Early Praise for *Beyond Disease Care*

I highly recommend this book as one of the best I have seen on educating people about the important differences between disease care and health care. The authors not only take a holistic approach on teaching us how to solve our chronic health conditions; they model that approach by combining the substantial medical knowledge of Walt Stoll with the cogent and articulate writing abilities of Kathleen Diehl. Rather than government legislation, this book would much better serve us in improving America's health-care problems.

~ Bill Manahan, MD
Past president of the American Holistic Medical Association,
Assistant professor at University of Minnesota

Dr. Walt Stoll's new book, *Beyond Disease Care,* is even better than his previous work, *Recapture Your Health,* and that is saying something. I especially praise Kathleen's straightforward writing style, which results in a very reader-friendly book that is also densely packed with useful information. Personally, I enjoyed his candid story of how he was pushed out of conventional medicine and instead, fortunately for all of us, championed natural health care. He is a strong critic of orthodox medicine, but his book offers the reader so much more than that: detailed, practical instruction on how to use natural treatment approaches to improve health. This is education, not medication, and I applaud it!

~ Andrew W. Saul, www.DoctorYourself.com
Editor of the Orthomolecular Medicine News Service,
Author of *Doctor Yourself* and *Fire Your Doctor!*

In an age of health care being defined as "managed" care, there needs to be a mutual participation between health-care provider and client in all aspects of treatment, recovery and prevention if we are to have a viable and sustainable health-care system. In truth, the role of a health-care provider should be—in the case of a client's dis-ease—to provide both necessary medicine and guidance so that, in the long run, the client is managing his or her own health. This is the goal of *Beyond Disease Care.*

I was privileged to work alongside Dr. Walt Stoll for six years and witness his caring genius. People came to him in all phases of stress and dis-ease. I witnessed those who would have otherwise gone from bad to worse improve dramatically and experience whole new levels of wellness. I also witnessed those who had come to the end of what conventional medical health care could offer them be revived by adopting Dr. Stoll's three-legged stool approach supplemented with his cutting edge wisdom of what medical science has to offer. A master clinician, he is truly the people's doctor.

Beyond Disease Care is for *everyone.* Regardless of how fantastic we may look and feel, all of us will experience various forms of sickness and distress over the course of our lives. And, we shall all grow old. Thus, if you are a patient who wants to "manage" the course of your own health and well-being or a health-care provider, be it conventional or alternative, you need this book as your companion. Use its wisdom alongside your own. And, when your clients are feeling so much better than they ever imagined or expected, make sure they get a copy of this book as well.

~ Robert Sachs
Social worker and massage therapist,
Author of *Tibetan Ayurveda*

As physicians we are trained to treat diseases and it seems the patient has been almost forgotten. Even our support groups support the disease not the person (cancer support group, epilepsy support group, etc.). In this remarkable book, Walt and Kathleen have given us an understanding of the difference between acute and chronic disease, and a deeper understanding of stress and how it affects the disease process. On top of that, they give us answers and ways in which we, as we take responsibility for our own care, can work with our health-care givers in attaining true healing, not just a cure. This book gives us many answers to our national health-care crisis. I highly recommend it to physicians and patients.

~ Gladys Taylor McGarey, MD, MD(H)
Past president of the American Holistic Medical Association,
Past president of Arizona Board of Homeopathic Medical Examiners

Seeing is believing. As a teenager, I watched in amazement as my father, Dr. Walt Stoll, actually de-aged himself. I literally saw the years, pounds and strain rapidly disappear from his body, mind and spirit. From there, I had an amazing bird's eye view as I witnessed this "founding father" use his open mind, keen intellect, amazing diagnostics skills and dedication to share his discoveries with patient after patient, many of whom were desperate in their search for help after being turned away from our traditional "disease-based" medical community. Finally, I watched him take his message to the world, teaching the powerful central tenets of holistic (complementary/integrative) medicine as described in *Beyond Disease Care*, his latest and best book.

Profoundly inspired, I spent fourteen years of my life studying osteopathic medicine and human physiology and then another sixteen years practicing medicine, teaching and conducting research related to the common sense of the holistic wisdom I learned from this pioneering physician. As a professional, I am indebted to my father for his dedication to health and the holistic medicine movement. As his son, I am inspired by my father's example of wisdom, courage, self-reliance, dedication, intellectual integrity, patience and service to others.

~ Scott T. Stoll, DO, PhD
Founding executive director, National Osteopathic Research Center
Former tenured professor, University of North Texas Health Science Center

If you want to take charge of your own health, read this book. The clear explanations of how health works and the many effective self-help tools will save you time, money and energy when working toward reversing your chronic health issues and optimizing your energy levels.

~ Jan DeCourtney, CMT
Holistic practitioner, owner of Life Spring Healing Arts
Co-author of *Recapture Your Health*

To Gloria -
Wishing you abundant health!
Kathleen

Beyond Disease Care

When Your TREATMENTS Fail to CURE You . . .

The Truth about How to Prevent and Reverse Today's Most Common Chronic Conditions

WALT STOLL, MD and KATHLEEN M. DIEHL

SUNRISE
HEALTH COACH
PUBLICATIONS
Boulder, Colorado

Disclaimer: The information contained within this book is for educational purposes only. It is not intended to prevent, diagnose, treat or cure any disease, and in no way constitutes medical advice. No claims, warranties or guarantees, expressed or implied, are being made about the ultimate safety and/or effectiveness of any of the information provided. You are hereby advised that the authors and publisher shall have neither liability nor responsibility to any person or entity with respect to any loss or damage caused, or alleged to be caused, directly or indirectly, by the use of any information contained within this book. Always consult a professional health practitioner both before and during the implementation of any new health regimen. *Never* discontinue any prescribed medication or treatment without first consulting the physician managing that treatment. Complementary medicine is just as its name implies—complementary to conventional medicine—not a replacement for it.

Publisher's Cataloging-in-Publication Data

Stoll, Walt.

Beyond disease care: when your treatments fail to cure you ... the truth about how to prevent and reverse today's most common chronic conditions / Walt Stoll and Kathleen Diehl.

p. cm.

Includes bibliographical references and index.

ISBN-13: 978-0-9653171-4-6 (alk. paper)

eBook ISBN-13: 978-0-9653171-8-4

1. Alternative Medicine—United States. 2. Diet—Health aspects. 3. Exercise—Health aspects. 4. Mind and Body. 5. Self-Care, Health.

I. Diehl, Kathleen. II. Title.

RA776.5 S859 2010

613—dc22 2010930628 CIP

Cover design by TLC Graphics, www.TLCGraphics.com.

Contact: The authors welcome your comments, constructive criticism and success stories. For book orders, media inquiries, wholesale ordering (including health-care practitioners interested in reselling *Beyond Disease Care*) and serial rights information, please visit the publisher's website.

SUNRISE HEALTH COACH PUBLICATIONS

Sunrise Health Coach Publications

for Stoll Foundation for Holistic Health

A project of United Charitable Programs, Inc., a registered 501(C)3 public charity

PO Box 21132

Boulder, CO 80308

www.sunrisehealthcoach.com

info@sunrisehealthcoach.com

To Jan DeCourtney,
whose experience, hard work and dedication
helped take our book through that final finish line.
Namaste to you!

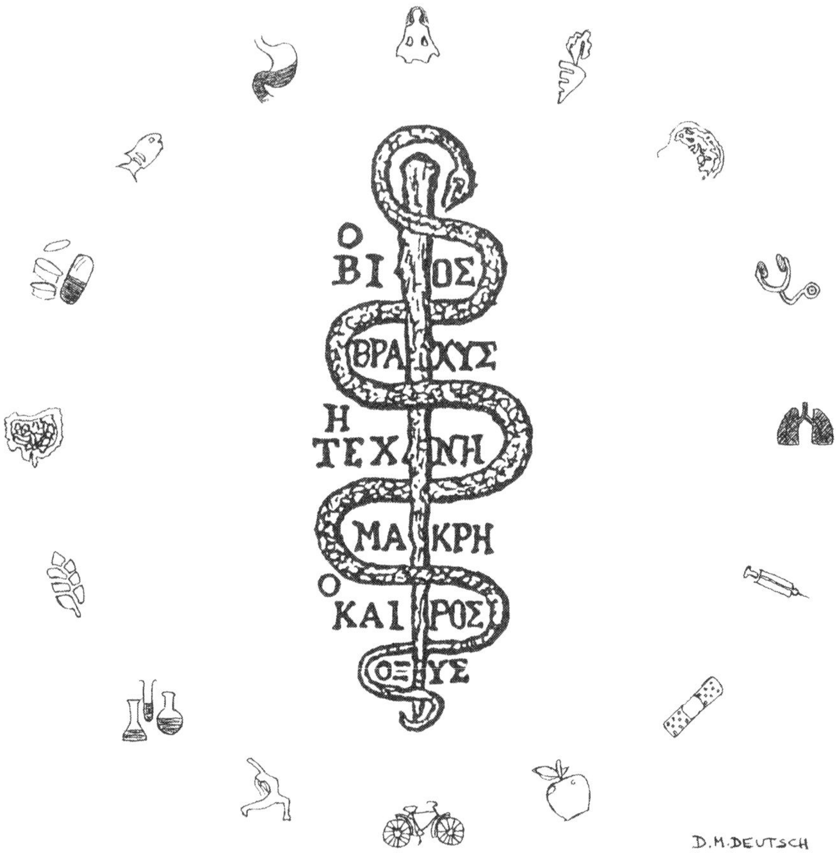

The Staff of Aesculapius

The Staff of Aesculapius

There was a time when becoming a healer was a "calling" with absolutely no monetary advantage. Healers such as shamans, medicine women and medicine men were at the apex or center of primitive society. The health and well-being of the patient was of primary importance. Unfortunately, the economic and political climate has changed the face of medicine. Somewhere along the line, a medical license became a ticket to great wealth, and the very word "healer" became unofficially synonymous with the word "quackery."

The words "holism" and "holy" both share the same root—"holos"—which means health. Every healing profession in the world (chiropractic, ayurveda, homeopathy, osteopathy, naturopathy, traditional Chinese medicine, etc.) *with the exception of allopathy* is based in a healthy lifestyle of exercise, relaxation and whole foods.

The vitalistic concept of health and wholeness was the basis for the original single snake emblem facing this page—the Staff of Aesculapius. Only within the past one hundred years has it been altered into the double snake caduceus representative of our current monopolistic disease-care system.

This ancient Staff of Aesculapius symbol represents where we came from, and the surrounding circle of icons represent the current importance of combining the best of *all* the world's healing philosophies. We offer this book as a comprehensive tool that you may use to create a reality of health and wholeness for yourself.

—Walt Stoll, MD

Contents

10. Recurrent Colds and Flu

11. Recurrent Ear Infections

12. Recurrent Headaches

13. Endocrine Disorders

14. Vascular Disorders

Section IV: The 3-Legged Stool (3LS) of Wellness

23. Introduction to the 3LS

24. Skilled Relaxation (The 1st Leg)

25. Aerobic Exercise (The 2nd Leg)

26. Whole Foods (The 3rd Leg)

Section V: Holistic Tools

27. Elimination/Provocation Diet

28. Intracellular Magnesium

29. Essential Fatty Acids

30. Avoiding Unnecessary Antibiotics

31. Hot Compresses

32. Gentle Rebounding

Charts, Figures & Illustrations

Foreword

by Robert Anderson, MD

When in the course of human evolution we undergo major paradigm shifts, significant dislocation and chaos is generally the result. Concepts upon which we were formerly dependent seem to pale in the light of new, unfamiliar ideas. Anchors to what we thought we knew as "truth" are suddenly lost, leaving us with a vague sense of uncertainty. We may feel adrift on a restless and stormy sea with no firm sense of direction—or worse—question our very survival along the shores of our newly shattered belief system.

This uncomfortable journey is called *progress*.

In recent decades, many of our important institutions have been passing through such a shift once again. None have been moving through the challenge of radical change with more distress than the professions involved with disease and healing.

Modern-day conventional medicine continues to embrace the monistic (singular) shore of Cartesian science. Clinging strongly to the concept of atomism with its pervasive emphasis on smaller and smaller segments of limited Western scientific ideas, conventional medicine's half-accurate point of view strongly resists our inevitable return to the vitalistic shore it has worked so hard to discredit. Vitalism encompasses the effective, thousand-year holistic healing traditions that honor the more natural, spiritual and ethereal aspects of health and well-being.

Over the past few centuries, innovative thinkers who have stepped forward with concepts that have fueled major shifts in the field of medicine have been vilified for the "radical" nature of their theories. For example, in the 1850s, obstetrician Ignaz Semmelweis was defamed by the medical establishment for correctly suggesting that contagion was responsible for the high death rate in women after childbirth. Yet when his followers began to assiduously cleanse their hands with soap and water between patients, mortality from postpartum fever fell from 18% down to only 1.2%. Semmelweis was severely criticized, portrayed as mad, forcibly restrained and finally incarcerated in an insane asylum, where he died. Twenty years later, his theories were accepted as factual by the medical community, and a monument in his honor was erected in Budapest.

In the nineteenth century, Louis Pasteur, physician and renowned developer of the germ theory of disease and the concepts of vaccination and pasteurization, engaged in public debate with physiologist Claude Bernard, champion of the concepts of homeostasis and immunity (or "territory" as first principle). Pasteur was said to have uttered on his deathbed: "Alas, Bernard was right, the germ is nothing—the milieu (the environment within) is everything." Pasteur lived as an atomist but died a vitalist.

Similarly, the late double Nobel Laureate Linus Pauling, PhD was severely criticized in the last half of the twentieth century for his ideas regarding the role of high-dose vitamin C in human health and disease, another vitalistic approach. As has been the pattern with all such historical medical paradigm shifts, numerous studies have since proven the pioneering thinker was right all along.

The well-known medical principle "do no harm" seems to have gotten lost by conventional medicine somewhere along the way. In fact, a 1998 review of 39 studies involving 153 hospitals estimated the U.S. in-patient death toll from prescription drugs, *appropriately used,* to be 106,000 per year. By 2004, a new study involving 37 million patient records determined there were 195,000 in-patient deaths per year due to preventable medical errors.[1]

In contrast, this very same "do no harm" principle has been honored throughout the ages and continues to be honored today by the many holistic, complementary and alternative approaches that are non-invasive, have practically no possibility of detriment and can often be instituted on a "why not?" basis.

With each passing year, more and more people are embracing vitalism as an indispensable component of this new shore of *Wellness.* Most of the tenets of this holistic paradigm are so basic and so self-evident that the thinking person must stop to question *why* conventional medicine continues its vehement resistance to validating their credibility. Sadly, the bottom line of their resistance is most often a political and financial one.

Despite conventional medicine's typical argument that alternative therapies are unsubstantiated and subject to suspicion, numerous holistic remedies have been systematically studied and the results, proving them safe and effective, widely published. The problem is, these types of studies are rarely being presented to students in U.S. conventional medical schools. The following are just two examples.

In 1985, the *Journal of the American Medical Association* (*JAMA*) published a controlled study in which 88% of patients with shingles (herpes zoster) were completely cured within three weeks of treatment with adenosine monophosphate (AMP) as compared to 43% of those treated with a placebo. AMP is a substance synthesized daily in the human body during normal metabolism. Even though the safety and efficacy of AMP is far better than drug treatments, conventional medicine continues its standard protocol of prescribing potent anti-virals, steroids, anti-seizure medications and narcotic pain pills as its treatment of choice.[2]

In another example, a nearly 50% reduction of blood loss during spinal surgery was achieved in a group of patients when it was suggested to them to "tell your blood to stay away from the site of the surgery during the operation and return afterward."[3] Since such a suggestion could never be harmful, why has this not become routine at every preoperative conference between patient and anesthesiologist? One conventional physician from an academic institution was quoted as saying, "Evidence for this [new] treatment is so preposterous that I wouldn't believe it even if it were true!"

The new wellness paradigm honors the ability of patients to to know—and ultimately *be responsible for*—their own minds and bodies. It demands a new openness on the part of conventional practitioners to abandon their narrow, restricted protocols and begin looking at a series of options not commonly considered. Finally, it calls for a shift toward the belief that exuberant health is possible for most of us.

Of the multitude of books available today on the topics of health and alternative medicine, I've yet to see one that gives as broad a picture, historically, politically and medically, without being the least bit boring. *Beyond Disease Care* explains not only *what* to do, but *why*—starting with a cutting-edge explanation of what "stress" really is. If you do nothing more than read about and embrace the three major lifestyle components of nutrition, exercise and relaxation as described, the undeniable increase in your health and well-being will be worth far more than the cover price.

This is the wonderful good news about the new paradigm espoused by Walt and Kathleen in this book. May you rediscover the art of wellness by utilizing the valuable information within.

~ Robert A. Anderson, MD
Co-Founder and Former President, American Holistic Medical Association
Founding President, American Board of Integrative Holistic Medicine

Preface

by Walt Stoll, MD

There is only one condition that is fatal 100% of the time. That condition is birth! No matter how healthy we may be or what preventives we may take, *none* of us will escape physical death. With that perspective in mind, the ultimate goal of the healing professions ought not to be avoidance of death, but *quality of life*.

DNA research has established that only 10–20% of diseases are due to our genetics (nature). The other 80–90% are due to a combination of environmental influences and our everyday lifestyle choices (nurture).[1] That means nurture is at least *four times* more important than nature—proving we as individuals have the power to prevent the vast majority of diseases. This is great news, because despite rapid advances in medical science we still have not mastered the technology to change our genetic defects. Until that day arrives, we would do well to make the best of whatever hand nature has dealt to each of us.

My own personal health challenges are a good example of the nature-nurture model. At the age of forty-five, I developed insulin-dependent type II diabetes. Identifying the genetic component wasn't difficult—*both* my parents had type II diabetes, and *all six* of my younger siblings have it. Furthermore, my own son developed type II diabetes in his twenties. In other words, nature strongly determined that I was likely to develop this condition—it was only a matter of *when*.

My discovery of the three-part health regimen known in this book as the "3-Legged Stool (3LS) of Wellness" predated the onset of my diabetes. New to the practice of medicine and wanting to set a good example for my patients, I began incorporating aerobic exercise into my lifestyle. I continued practicing aerobics for ten years, with wonderful results, before discovering that changing my eating habits would greatly *multiply* those wonderful results. The better I felt, the more I found myself motivated to learn and practice additional health-promoting habits, including specific relaxation techniques such as meditation and massage. With each of these three lifestyle changes—aerobic exercise, a healthful diet and effective relaxation techniques—I experienced a quantum leap in my health and well-being.

Chapter 2 describes the multitude of chronic health conditions I myself was suffering before discovering and implementing the lifestyle practices just mentioned. Not only did I quickly recover from my long list of health complaints, I also greatly *delayed* the inevitable onset of my type II diabetes. After its onset, the 3LS of Wellness gave me a much higher quality of life than I would have otherwise had. It also prevented and/or delayed many of diabetes' serious secondary complications.

Eventually some damaging effects did occur, beginning with a few transient ischemic attacks (TIAs) and my first coronary in 2003. However, I've remained free of some of the most devastating complications such as diabetic peripheral neuropathy, loss of circulation to my limbs and resulting amputation. In fact, all my doctors and specialists are amazed at how long I have lived and how healthy I have remained. By all their estimations, I should have been dead at least ten years ago.

I attribute my success to a combination of the 3LS lifestyle, holistic therapies such as those presented in this book, and yes, various conventional treatments. Given some of the topics covered here, people sometimes get the false impression that I'm against all conventional medicine. Nothing could be further from the truth. I've learned that the best of both worlds lies in combining alternatives *with* conventional medicine—now usually termed "integrative medicine." I can't over-emphasize this point enough: Complete health care must include both conventional medicine *and* alternative approaches, not either/or!

This practical and candidly thought-provoking book offers over five decades of my personal and professional knowledge and experience. It also documents—in a clear and concise manner—*how* and *why* our country is in the midst of a serious disease-care crisis. Thanks to my co-authoring partnership with Kathleen, the teachings I've been offering throughout the years are now compiled and written in this organized, engaging, and easy-to-understand book, giving you a leg up on what I had to learn the hard way.

Remember, we all shall die in the end! Think of this book as a tool for adding years to your life—and life to your years. Namaste!

~ Walt Stoll, MD
Author, *Saving Yourself from the Disease-Care Crisis*
Co-author, *Recapture Your Health*
www.askwaltstollmd.com

Introduction

by Kathleen M. Diehl

"If you have these questions, then so must many others." These words, typed by Walt Stoll, MD in response to one of my initial posts to his online bulletin board over a decade ago, were the very words that first intrigued and inspired me to want to learn more about what this outspoken, progressive physician had to say. It didn't take long for me to realize I had stumbled upon something very rare, indeed.

Here was this experienced and knowledgeable medical doctor who was willing, not only to truly *listen* to me, but to take the time to answer my personal health questions from an entirely new perspective. Unlike the "Doctor as God" dynamic under which I'd been raised, here was a doctor who challenged me to examine my life-long illusions about health and dis-ease (hyphenated to illustrate the word's true meaning). When I first found Dr. Stoll's website, I was so left-brained in my thinking that getting me to see beyond my conditioned viewpoints was no easy task.

Dr. Stoll (or "Walt," as his patients and friends call him) not only taught me new ways of looking at *why* the conventional approach alone had failed to cure my chronic conditions, he also held me accountable for my own health. I was in for a huge wake-up call, to say the least. From one light-bulb moment to the next, I found myself embarking on an incredible journey of releasing my former false notions about treatments, cures and how to be healthy. As of this book's original printing, Walt still gives of his time answering the thousands of questions posed to him via his online bulletin board, free of charge, just as he has done since 1996.[1]

Many of the questions posed online were from people who had read his first book, *Saving Yourself from the Disease-Care Crisis,* and wanted to learn more.[2] Based on public demand, his website grew into a treasure trove of information, much of it buried in its vast archives of questions and answers covering over 270 topics. Several participants began asking, "Walt, any plans for a new, more expansive book?" The growing need for such a book was obvious, and I felt very drawn to get involved.

Ever since I can remember, I've been attracted to researching health and medical topics. By the age of fourteen, I was already reading up on the then-new theories of antioxidants and free radicals! It's no wonder I was interested, because throughout my youth I suffered severe allergies and asthma, as well as back-to-back respiratory tract infections including colds, flu, bronchitis, sinusitis, strep throat, ear infections and pneumonia. I also had frequent migraines and bouts with what my mother called the "stomach flu."

Once I reached adulthood, my asthma mostly resolved but I continued to struggle with a variety of health challenges. As time went on, I found myself being diagnosed with more and more "new" conditions, including menorrhagia (with resulting chronic anemia), fibrocystic breast disease, a pituitary prolactinoma, osteopenia (discovered after I broke my hip from a simple fall at age 26), arthritis and tendonitis, degenerative discs in my neck, fibromyalgia, autoimmune thyroid disease (including three thyroid tumors), neurocardiogenic syncope (a form of dysautonomia), kidney stones and, and, and ... I think you get the idea. I have spent more hours in doctors' and specialists' waiting rooms than I care to admit. Well, nothing sparks interest quite like necessity.

Added to this equation was a deep fascination about the interconnectedness of body, mind and spirit and a strong passion for writing. My desire to do something big with these combined interests was growing. I assumed Walt was joking when he said he was looking for someone to help write his next book, at which point I (not jokingly) said, "I will!" Thus, our co-authoring partnership began.

I think it important now to anticipate and address a likely question in your mind, various versions of which I've heard before: "How are you, having had no formal medical training whatsoever, qualified to write a book of this nature?" (Hey, it's a valid question!) Ironically, the beauty of our co-authoring partnership lies in the very fact that I am *not* a doctor. Instead, I represent all the people who've spent years trying to solve their own chronic health complaints through the system as it stands—learning firsthand the ineffectiveness (and sometimes danger) of believing treatment-based approaches would actually *cure* the majority of what ailed them.

Beyond Disease Care has been a joint project in which each author has played very different roles. Walt's roles include doctor and teacher. He is the one with the conventional medical degree, the post-graduate training in numerous holistic practices, and the years of experience that form the basis for what lies within. Everything included in this book has received the careful scrutiny and, I assure you, the final approval of this highly educated and experienced physician.

My roles in this co-authoring partnership include writer and editor, researcher and organizer. But perhaps more importantly, like a foreign language interpreter, I seek to bridge the gap between doctors and patients. After all, how many of us have resigned ourselves to (or worse, lived to regret) taking our doctor's word for everything without doing our own research or listening to our own gut feelings? How many of us are seeking relief from the prescription pad without understanding what we're really getting, or *risking*? Too few of us have been raised to listen to our own bodies or trust our own intuition—especially those who, like me, were brought up to view doctors (and religion) as authorities not to be questioned and certainly not to be challenged.

What I first thought would take me about a year or two to accomplish ended up becoming an increasingly (even embarrassingly) long journey of study, research, organization, writing and re-writing. As I e-mailed and phoned Walt with questions that came to mind along the way, he consistently and patiently responded with his answers. If I still did not fully grasp a concept, I asked follow-up questions until it was made clear. After all, if I didn't understand something, then I couldn't very well write about it in a way that our readers would understand it.

As my perception of what truly constitutes an infallible recipe for a healthy, joyous life continues to grow and evolve, I have come to view Walt's teachings as a springboard or bridge builder for expanding awareness and questioning *all* concepts formerly accepted as truths. In the body-mind-spirit trinity, I believe that when we can connect with the Self as spirit *first*, our minds and bodies naturally follow suit. For some, this book will be about "doing," following processes and guidelines that lead toward health. For others, this book will be about "being," creating a sense of inner freedom where before there may have been a sense of bondage.

It's time to become an active participant in your own health care. I invite you join the thousands of citizens who are awakening to a larger truth and put the ultimate responsibility for your own well-being into the only hands where it rightfully belongs—your own. Whether or not you take action on the concepts contained within, you will be empowered by at least *knowing* that you do, indeed, have that choice if and when you decide you are ready to embrace it. I wish you many blessings on your journey to abundant health.

~ Kathleen M. Diehl
Author: *The Collective Awakening*
www.thecollectiveawakening.com
www.kathleendiehl.com

How to Use This Book

IMPORTANT! There are five sections in this book. Each chapter in the first two sections successively builds upon the information in the last, forming the basis for understanding the final three sections. Just as you cannot expect to build a sturdy house without first laying its foundation, so too, you cannot expect to gain a sturdy understanding of the last half of this book without first laying *its* foundation. While it may be tempting to flip to Section III: *Chronic Health Conditions* right away (especially when you see one or more that you've been dealing with), to do so without taking the time to read the first two sections would be to do yourself a great disservice.

Section I: *Laying the Foundation* does exactly what its name suggests, laying the necessary foundation or groundwork for the remainder of the book. Explore the differences between conventional medicine and the world's many other healing philosophies and enjoy a brief summary of the historical events that led to our country's profit-based monopolistic system of medicine and its resulting disease-care crisis.

Section II: *Precursors to Chronic Health Conditions* builds upon the foundation laid in the first section, taking you on a fascinating journey into the *how* and *why* behind the development of chronic dis-ease. Redefine the word "stress" and discover how accumulated stress-effect storage in the hypothalamus is the true root cause of nearly all chronic and degenerative conditions so prevalent in our fast-paced, high-tech society.

Section III: *Chronic Health Conditions* delves into many of today's most common chronic conditions, comparing conventional medical approaches with those of holistic medicine. Break free from the many illusions inherent in our country's disease-care mentality by learning specific complementary treatments you can safely try at home. The chapters in this section can be read in any order.

Section IV: ***The 3-Legged Stool (3LS) of Wellness*** outlines the three most important Wellness practices proven to prevent and/or reverse chronic disease: Skilled Relaxation, Aerobic Exercise and Whole Foods.* This is the action-based portion of the book—the real, long-term formula for how to be healthy—and, by far, the most important to heed.

Section V: ***Holistic Tools*** provides detailed instructions for the specific holistic suggestions that are recommended throughout Sections III and IV. Although none of these tools will interfere with any conventional treatment you may be taking, *never* discontinue any prescribed treatment without the advice and supervision of a qualified medical professional.

And finally, the book concludes with a helpful three-part **Appendix,** a list of **Endnotes** for references and resources cited, a **Glossary** for defining frequently-used terms and a detailed **Index** for quickly finding the page number(s) of any topic that interests you.

As explained in the Introduction, this book came about through a collaborative partnership between doctor (Walt) and lay person (Kathleen), designed to bridge the communication gap between physicians and their patients. Every effort has been made to provide cutting-edge information that is both useful and informative, while at the same time keeping that information simple enough to demystify all things "medical" and engaging enough to happily keep your attention.

Think of *Beyond Disease Care* as an invaluable and timeless owner's manual for your body; one which you will find yourself referring to both now and in the years to come. Let the journey begin …

---

* Note: The term "Wellness," along with its 3LS constituents, "Skilled Relaxation," "Aerobic Exercise" and "Whole Foods," will be capitalized throughout this book for emphasis. For additional information and comprehensive support with implementing the 3LS, read *Recapture Your Health* by Walt Stoll, MD and Jan DeCourtney, CMT.

Section I

LAYING THE FOUNDATION

The Conventional Medical Monopoly
(and How It Perpetuates Itself)

CHAPTER I

Health Care or *Disease* Care?

Truth passes through three stages before it is recognized.
In the first it is ridiculed; in the second it is opposed;
in the third it is regarded as self-evident.

~ Arthur Schopenhauer
(German philosopher, 1788–1860)

Sick and Tired (of Being Sick and Tired)

What you are holding in your hands is the culmination of my life's work of over fifty years as a medical doctor and health educator. I trust you will find the information within these pages eye opening, life changing, fun to read and easy to understand.* This book is designed to provide a foundation of knowledge upon which you may build for yourself a future of improved health and quality of life. I know of no other book on the market today that provides a more relevant big picture of the *how* and *why* behind modern-day chronic disease, and no other book that offers the wide assortment of safe and effective alternatives that can be tried in addition to any conventional treatments you may already be using.

I will begin by making important distinctions between conventional (allopathic) and alternative philosophies; including describing the vital differences between acute and chronic health conditions, treatments and cures, health care and disease care. Without this foundational understanding, trying to figure out the best approach for your individual condition(s) is not only confusing, but misleading.

* Reminder: The words "I," "me" and "my" throughout this book refer only to Dr. Stoll.

What Is . . . ?

- **Conventional Medicine:** An atomistic healing philosophy that operates as a powerful functional monopoly in the United States. Its emphasis is on diagnosing and treating the *symptoms* of disease, rather than preventing and reversing the *causes*. Also known as "allopathic medicine."
- **Allopathic Medicine/Allopathy:** The original term for "conventional medicine."
- **Homeopathic Medicine/Homeopathy:** The healing approach of administering an extremely diluted amount of the same substance that is believed to be causing the illness ("like cures like"). Homeopathy is one of the dominant healing philosophies in most of the world, and is the official healing philosophy of the British royal family.
- **Alternative Medicine:** A general term referring to any healing philosophy or technique other than conventional medicine.
- **Complementary Medicine:** Alternative medicine used in conjunction with (as a complement to) conventional medicine.
- **Holistic Medicine:** A vitalistic healing philosophy that emphasizes viewing the patient as a whole, focusing on patient education, personal responsibility and lifestyle to achieve balance and well-being. Holistic medicine, by definition, encompasses the effective elements of *all* the world's healing philosophies, including conventional medicine. Currently also becoming known as "integrative medicine."

Perhaps the readers who stand to benefit the most from this book are those who have reached the point of being "sick and tired of being sick and tired." Unfortunately, that's often what it takes for so many of us to become ready to move beyond the mindset of simply *covering up our symptoms* with various medical treatments. Suffering can be a blessing in disguise, providing the incentive and motivation to start taking personal responsibility for our own health and well-being.

I offer a unique perspective that can only come from having been on both sides of the medical fence, both professionally *and* personally. I went from practicing (and teaching) strictly conventional medicine to becoming so impressed by the results of alternative approaches that I slowly began incorporating these *complementary* principles into my practice.

As Chapter 2 will detail, for reasons that had absolutely nothing to do with my competency as a physician, incorporating alternatives into my practice led to an unfortunate series of harassments and eventually cost me my medical license. Despite this devastating loss, nothing could take from me the knowledge and experience I had gained from having already applied the principles—and experienced the benefits—of both conventional *and* complementary approaches. I had seen the strengths and weaknesses of each. I had witnessed the startling turnarounds, not only in my own chronic conditions, but in my patients' as well. I had also seen the hunger of my community for the information being denied them by our country's one-sided, profit-driven approach to disease.

The purpose of this book is three-fold: to educate the public about the "health-care" system as it stands; to bring back an appreciation for the value of the world's many effective holistic approaches; and to empower you, the reader, with the information you've likely been missing when it comes to solving your own chronic health conditions. I believe the first step toward fulfilling that purpose is a willingness to call our current system of medicine exactly what it is—"disease care." To understand what is meant by this unusual terminology, we will begin by exploring the crutial difference between *acute* and *chronic* health conditions, as well as the difference between a *treatment* and a *cure*.

Acute Versus Chronic

An "acute" health condition can be defined as any illness or set of symptoms that comes on suddenly and tends to be short lived. Examples include various injuries (such as broken bones, burns and skin wounds), food poisoning, accidental overdoses, appendicitis, acute infections and so forth. Most acute health conditions are generally well-managed by conventional treatment options. In fact, every year people from all over the world come to the United States seeking effective and even life-saving treatments for what conventional medicine is best at solving—acute conditions like trauma and infectious disease.

In contrast, a "chronic" health condition can be defined as any illness or set of symptoms that develops slowly over time, remains persistent or tends to recur. Examples of some of today's most common chronic health conditions (many of which were practically unheard of just a century ago) include depression, anxiety disorders, insomnia, allergies, eczema, environmental sensitivities, asthma, migraine headaches, thyroid disorders, hormonal imbalances, arthritis, fibromyalgia, adult acne, diabetes, obesity, chronic fatigue syndrome, hypertension, heart disease, cancer, gastrointestinal disturbances and immune system disorders (*not* an all-inclusive list). These days, it's hard to find *anyone* who isn't suffering from at least one variation of these types of conditions.

Keep in mind that some acute conditions can also be considered chronic if an individual repeatedly suffers one episode after the other. Examples in this book include the common cold, headaches and ear infections.

Chronic conditions continue to emerge in record numbers throughout the population and are therefore the focus of this book. With an estimated 133 million people suffering from chronic conditions in the United States alone, this category accounts for a whopping 85% of the complaints seen in family practice clinics today.[1]

When you add to this equation society's convenience-at-all-costs mentality, you find each new generation paying a greater price. Already, sedentary children raised on refined diets are becoming obese and acquiring serious chronic diseases at younger ages than ever before. As if that weren't enough, our society is being perpetually conditioned to seek cures where cures cannot be found. Unlike acute conditions, most chronic conditions are neither cured nor well managed by conventional treatment options. Instead, this category is best approached by all the other globally practiced paradigms that have both prevention *and* health promotion (Wellness) as their mainstays.*

---

* Reminder: Throughout the book, the word "Wellness" will be capitalized for emphasis, as will its three constituents: "Skilled Relaxation (SR)," "Aerobic Exercise" and "Whole Foods." To understand *why* Wellness works to reverse chronic disease, see Section II: *Precursors to Chronic Health Conditions.* To learn *how* to incorporate Wellness into your everyday life, see Section IV: *The 3-Legged Stool of Wellness.*

The truth is, no singular healing approach works (or is even appropriate) for all conditions. Just as thousands of people from other countries travel to the United States each year seeking the very best conventional medical has to offer, so too, thousands of people (with the financial luxury to do so) travel *out of* the United States each year in search of holistic solutions to their chronic and degenerative conditions—the category our incomplete system consistently fails to resolve. This leads us to another vital concept: There is a big difference between a "treatment" and a "cure." These two words are *not* synonymous!

Treatment Versus Cure

Diagnoses, by their very nature, are educated guesses and are far from infallible. Once a diagnosis is made, conventional medical treatments typically include one of two things: surgery (often preventable, unnecessary and/or harmful) and/or prescription medications (ditto). When it comes to chronic conditions, most treatments are simply suppressive therapies designed to provide relief by *masking your symptoms.* Your doctor knows these suppressive therapies won't cure you but is unlikely to explain this unless *you* bring it up.

Here are some common examples of the conventional treatment approach to chronic conditions. If you are in pain, the doctor prescribes pain medications to help reduce inflammation and/or suppress the pain signals coming from your brain. If you suffer from allergies, the doctor prescribes antihistamines to help suppress the histamine reactions of your immune system. If depressed, antidepressant medication may be prescribed to inhibit the reuptake of serotonin by the neurons in your central nervous system. Sound familiar?

Although there is no denying some level of relief is usually obtained, such symptom-suppressing medications should be thought of for exactly what they are—*treatments,* not *cures.* If the symptoms of a particular condition require repeated doctor visits and ongoing treatment, or, if symptoms return soon after treatment is discontinued, this certainly could not be considered a cure. People who trust the plethora of pharmaceutical advertisements as their main authority on how to approach health and disease could live their whole lives with no awareness of this simple truth.

Since most conventional treatments can do nothing about *why* you developed the condition in the first place, most can do nothing to prevent the condition (and all its accompanying symptoms) from continuing or returning in the future. The wisest healers know that chronic health conditions are not caused by a deficiency of the drugs used to treat them. As I've always said, "The resolution of chronic health problems will never come from something you *take*, but from something you *do*." Despite any improvement you may enjoy while on your medication(s), if you aren't simultaneously addressing the underlying root cause of your particular condition(s), your symptoms can be expected to continue—and progress—unabated.

What, then, is a cure? A true cure, by definition, means your body has returned to its normal, healthy, pre-disease function and no longer requires treatment. With a cure, you basically go on with your life as if nothing ever happened. Although conventional medicine is capable of curing certain *acute* conditions, when it comes to the majority of our *chronic* conditions, what it has to offer is more along the lines of disease management. Indeed, once a disease has progressed to the point of being irreversible, such an offering may well be necessary.

The conventional medical system is set up for the diagnosis and treatment of *disease*, not for the prevention of disease or the promotion of *health*. That is why I believe "disease care" is a far more accurate term for what U.S. citizens are actually getting. We have been conditioned to call it "health care" for political and economic reasons, not because that's what it truly is.

This bears repeating: While conventional medicine shines in so many important areas, it can offer *no cure* for the vast majority of chronic health conditions so prevalent in modern-day society. I know this may come as a shock to suffering patients who have been under the impression that a cure is what they were getting inside their prescription bottles. The truth is, many conventional treatments actually *expand* disease.[2]

Whatever Happened to "First, Do No Harm"?

Physicians entering the practice of medicine have taken various versions of the so-called "Hippocratic Oath" for about 2,000 years. Most people associate the Hippocratic Oath with the classic phrase, "First, do no harm." Although this exact wording never actually appeared in the oath, the phrase became popular because it embodied the most important theme of Hippocrates' teachings.[3]

When I took the oath back in 1962, "First, do no harm" was still the prominent theme by which medicine was to be practiced, reminding us physicians that the patients' best interests must always come first. The version I took had its graduates affirming: "I will follow that system of regimen which, according to my ability and judgment, I consider for the benefit of my patients, and abstain from whatever is deleterious and mischievous."[4]

Today, many contemporary medical schools impose a revised, modernized version of the oath as an admonition and affirmation to which their graduating classes assent. The new (AMA-approved) version of the oath has graduates reciting: "I will be loyal to the profession of medicine and just and generous to its members."[5] To whose benefit is the oath's admonition now?

More and more people are awakening to the fact that our disease-care system is indeed operating under powerful, profit-driven motives. Yet others remain oblivious. Until I *personally* experienced otherwise, I had no idea that the system to which I had dedicated my professional life had any ulterior motives. I was also completely unaware of the 2,500 year-old philosophical controversy regarding what should constitute the basis for our country's healing professions—atomism or vitalism.

Atomism: An Allopathic Paradigm

On one side of this historical controversy were the *atomists*, who held that the human bodymind is basically nothing more than a machine in which tiny particles get combined and recombined. Atomism is the philosophical basis for the allopathic paradigm as we know it today. The atomists believed if we could just break each function of the human body down into small enough units, we would eventually be able to solve its mystery and control its every aspect.[6]

In colonial times, Dr. Benjamin Rush (co-signer of the Declaration of Independence) came down firmly on the side of atomism, thus starting U.S. allopathic medicine on the path it continues to follow to this day. He was quoted as saying, "Although a certain self-acting power does exist in the organism, it is subject to ordinary physical and chemical laws and, in any case, it is not strong enough to withstand the onslaughts of disease."[7]

At the turn of the twentieth century, Sir William Osler, MD (co-founding professor of Johns Hopkins University), also enunciated the current atomistic paradigm of medical care when he stated: "The body has no way to prevent disease. It just happens to us. The only rational purpose of medicine is to diagnose the disease and do the best we can to alleviate symptoms."[8] Unfortunately, because it serves the *system* so nicely, our approach to health care is still operating under this hundred-year-old fallacy.

Vitalism: A Holistic Paradigm

On the opposite side of this historical controversy were the *vitalists*, who held that the human bodymind has a self-healing capacity within and a natural ability to protect itself from environmental degradations, illness and aging. The vitalists believed that a healer's efforts were best focused on removing interferences to health. The idea was to support the bodymind while allowing its innate intelligence to do its thing. All healing philosophies in the world today, except allopathy, are based in vitalism.

Hippocrates was the first recorded vitalist, which happens to be the philosophy most in alignment with "First, do no harm." Even back in his day, the wisest physicians knew that nature did most of the healing, and that only the proper management of the underlying causes behind the symptoms could ever truly prevent, treat or cure disease.

Every historical account of medicine that I've ever read acknowledges this division of thought between the atomists and the vitalists. One excellent resource for delving deeper is *Planet Medicine* by Richard Grossinger, PhD; another, the 2,200-page, four-volume *Divided Legacy* by Harris L. Coulter, PhD.[9] Authored by the world's foremost medical anthropologists, both works describe the progression of all the world's healing philosophies from 3,500 years ago to the present, tracing this debate through every era of history. Both were uncannily accurate with their predictions about what we are now experiencing politically, and both do a decent job of illustrating what we can expect in the future.

Another simple and concise publication for understanding the history of the philosophical conflicts that led to our current disease-care crisis is *Pigs in the Dirt* by Dean Black, PhD. In only seventy pages of text, followed by seventy pages of notes and quotes, he clearly documents how we got into such a mess and what we are going to have to do to get ourselves out of it. He goes even deeper into the issues in his other book, *Health at the Crossroads,* which in my opinion, should be required reading for every legislator in our country.[10]

Holism: A Merging of Philosophies

The debate between the atomists and the vitalists is reminiscent of the debate in particle physics that began in the 1600s. The controversy centered around whether light behaved like a wave, or like a particle. The physicists on the side of the wave theory did experiments proving that light, indeed, behaved like a wave. The physicists on the side of the particle theory also did experiments proving that light, indeed, behaved like a particle. The debate was finally resolved in the 1920s when both sides realized and agreed that light behaves both like a wave *and* like a particle.[11]

The opposite of a correct statement is a false statement.
But the opposite of a profound truth may well be another profound truth.

~ Niels Bohr (1885–1962)

Our current medical debate could be resolved by each side acknowledging that both atomism *and* vitalism are valid (albeit individually crippled) philosophies. The vitalists have been willing to co-exist for over a generation, but for political and economic reasons, the atomists would seemingly rather live with the consequences of their continued denial. Since practically none of the chronic conditions so widespread today were commonly seen in Dr. Rush's day (early 1800s), our continued reliance on the atomistic philosophy alone is not only extremely outdated but outrageously inappropriate.

When I was in medical school, our one and only medical history course was taught by an allopath whose curriculum included only the history of allopathy. Since nothing based on vitalism was ever mentioned, the pervasive impression and resulting collective assumption we emerged with was that only the *allopathic* philosophy was truly valid. When I later discovered and began incorporating alternatives into my practice, I had no idea I was combining two halves of an ancient debate. All I knew was how much better my patients did with this expanded approach. Instead of viewing vitalistic philosophies as *competition*, it became obvious to me that they were *complementary* to my conventional offerings.

Our health-care battle is no longer based on scientific debate. It is now based, almost completely, on economic and political power. The present disease-care crisis is the result, and we citizens are the casualties.[12] Only through public education can we ever hope to move from our current system of profit-driven disease care to an effective system of patient-driven health care. Truly, the accumulated burdens of modern-day life have created a world in which humans no longer thrive (or sometimes even survive) with either philosophy alone.

The word "holistic" means "the whole." We are more than just our bodies—we are body, mind and spirit. Holism takes into account the whole person, and holistic medicine, by definition, encompasses the effective elements of *all* the world's healing philosophies—including conventional medicine.

CHAPTER 2

From Conventional to Holistic: How I Lost My License

Someone must teach new things. Someone must take the abuse. Someone must be ostracized. Someone must be called a fraud and a quack. Then, out of all of it, comes the new truth to become a part of us.

~ Fred Hart
(Founder of the National Health Federation, 1888–1975)

Who *Is* Walt Stoll?

For anyone who would like to know more about who I am and how I came to know and teach the principles in this book, this chapter contains somewhat of a professional autobiography. Yet it is more than just *my* story, it is a story representative of so many of my colleagues—and of the flaws inherent in our disease-care system. I wish I could say that scenarios such as what I am about to describe are completely a thing of the past. Although we've come a long way in the decades since I first entered practice, we still have a very long way to go.

I graduated from high school in 1954, earned my bachelor's degree in psychology in 1958, then graduated from Ohio State University with my MD in 1962. After completing my internship in 1963, I spent the next ten years as a board-certified family practitioner in a small rural community in Ohio. The following three years, I was an instructor at the University of Kentucky School of Allied Health, where I had a joint appointment as assistant professor of medicine in the Department of Family Practice at the University of Kentucky School of Medicine.

In 1976, I founded the Holistic Medical Centre in Lexington, Kentucky. I was its director until 1989, at which point I moved into solo family practice of Wellness Medicine in Nicholasville, Kentucky. I remained in practice there until 1993. The last seventeen years of my thirty-year career were spent practicing holistic medicine; that is, conventional medicine used in conjunction with as many alternative and complementary healing approaches as I could possibly learn.* This combination is now commonly referred to as "integrative medicine."

Complete Life Transformation

In 1976, while still an instructor at the University of Kentucky School of Allied Health, I was officially introduced to the world of holistic medicine. During a course in applied kinesiology (known as "AK" or "muscle testing") taught by Michael Lerner, DMD, I witnessed a demonstration that convinced me of something never mentioned in any of my conventional training—sugar was damaging my health! Believe it or not, this concept was quite novel to me at the time.

When I first met Dr. Lerner, I was suffering from several chronic health conditions as well as a lifelong weight problem, weighing in at 242 pounds. I was under the treatment of three separate allopathic specialists: a surgeon for my hemorrhoids as well as the bulging discs in my back; an internist for my chronic indigestion, sinusitis and arthritis as well as my dangerously high cholesterol (over 300) and resulting hypertension (160/110); and last but not least, a psychiatrist for my chronic depression and insomnia.

At the time, my prescription drugs included Talwin for pain, Valium for muscle tension, Quaalude for insomnia, Mylanta and Probanthine for indigestion and Elavil for depression—all at the same time. I was confined to wearing a back brace and had been told that the only potential solutions to my miserable state included various surgical procedures

* For a more detailed account of Walt's professional history and his full curriculum vitae, including primary, graduate and post-graduate education, professional history, board certifications, society memberships, major workshops and presentations, media events, publications and major public service contributions, please go to http://askwaltstollmd.com/book_author_cv_walt.shtml.

and life-long prescription drugs. Of course, I went along with it because this was exactly the type of advice I'd been giving my own patients. *It was all I knew!*

Dr. Lerner recommended a Whole Foods diet, which I somewhat skeptically agreed to follow on a two-week trial basis. Skeptical because, like so many people in the '70s, I had no idea that processed food could be affecting my health. For the sake of convenience (and given the long list of potentially hidden ingredients to avoid), I chose to eat nothing but brown rice topped with steamed vegetables. I kept up my previously established routine of Aerobic Exercise three times per week, and in addition, began practicing Silva Mind Training—one of the many forms of Skilled Relaxation (SR).[1] Little did I know this would mark the beginning of a *complete life transformation.*

So dramatic was my improvement in those first two weeks, I had more than enough incentive to keep going. Within six months of following this lifestyle protocol, later renamed the 3-Legged Stool (3LS) of Wellness, my long list of symptoms had abated and I was safely off all my medications. As an added bonus, I noticed I was no longer catching nearly every cold and flu from my patients because my immune system had become so strong. Feeling better than I ever had in my entire life, I was utterly *brimming* with enthusiasm about my new "discovery."

Of course, my patients noticed the dramatic change and started asking me what in the world I'd been doing to get so much healthier in such a short period of time. That's when it hit me—I really didn't understand the details about *how* and *why* these three lifestyle methods worked. All I knew was that when I followed this lifestyle protocol every day for six months, *I became well.*

Prior to this experience, conventional medicine was the only healing modality I considered valid. Then it hit me. I was standing at a major crossroads in my professional life. I could either look the other way (continue the protocol of giving patients the conventional treatments they thought they wanted, whether it hurt them or not) *and become a rich man,* or I could be honest with my patients about the necessity of adopting a Wellness lifestyle *and risk losing them to the physician down the street.* For me, the decision was obvious.

I decided to enroll in post-graduate training—this time, in a variety of alternative healing approaches—while simultaneously keeping up with the latest in conventional medicine. Although I found myself putting in longer hours than ever before, my enthusiasm for discovering more about the world's time-tested, "unconventional" healing philosophies gave me boundless energy. That very same year, I gradually assembled a well-rounded team of holistic professionals and founded the Holistic Medical Centre in Lexington, Kentucky.

The Birth of My Holistic Medical Centre

My staff included a chiropractor; an applied kinesiology practitioner (who also incorporated herbology and aromatherapy); a Chinese medicine practitioner (who was also an expert in macrobiotics, reflexology, acupressure and several forms of therapeutic massage); a holistic dentist with expertise in removing mercury-containing dental amalgams (who also specialized in temperomandibular joint dysfunction, homeopathy, electromagnetic medical diagnosis and therapy and electroacupuncture); a chaplain with a master's degree in counseling (who was also an expert in biofeedback and the teaching of SR techniques); and a certified physician's assistant (who graduated from the clinical associate program at the University of Kentucky School of Allied Health, a curriculum developed by myself). In addition, a naturopathic physician from the community was brought in as needed for cooperative consultation. I provided the allopathic medical portion—still my area of expertise and the best approach for some conditions.

As the Centre's director, it was also my job to integrate the team's recommendations. Each new patient received a detailed 75-page "New Patient Handbook." This handbook gradually grew to cover much of what you will find in the three-part Appendix at the back of this book.[2] It wasn't long before our reputation attracted patients from around the world, from China to the Bahamas, some presenting with the most complicated of cases. Meeting this challenge necessitated our developing a very creative approach. We decided to set aside one day a week in which a small group of such patients would receive the attention of the entire medical staff.

Our "Thursday Clinic"

Every Thursday, on a rotating basis, these complex patients would receive a one-hour consultation with each and every professional on the team. Since this process took the entire day, the staff would bring in various Whole Foods dishes to share as a potluck lunch. This not only demonstrated to the patients how delicious and satisfying a perfect diet could be, it also allowed us all to spend time socializing on equal ground. After all the consultations were complete, the staff would gather to present and compare our individual findings and recommendations with one another. We would finally finish around 8:00 p.m., exhausted but fulfilled by the intensity of what we learned that day and excited about what was being accomplished for these particular patients.

Our composite evaluation detailed the following, each in order of their significance: a list of the patients' diagnoses; a list of the suspected causes; our recommendations for solutions that would produce the best results with the least amount of time, effort and expense; and finally, our observations of the patients' strengths and available resources for implementing our proposals. The following morning, with the typed reports in hand, I'd spend an additional hour with each patient presenting the team's consensus and answering any questions. They were then sent on their way with an audio recording of the entire appointment (something we were already in the habit of doing for all our routine office patients).

Profits took a hit with this approach, but somehow that didn't seem to matter. We found ourselves rewarded with those "treasures more precious than gold" mentioned in the Bible. The excellent camaraderie and excitement of our teamwork approach left us all quite happy and satisfied. Not only were we learning a great deal from one another about our respective professions but, more importantly, our most challenging patients were enjoying remarkable results.

Simple logic tells you that the faster patients can be escorted in and out of the exam room, the more money the system stands to make. This is not meant to imply that individual doctors do business with those intentions. Most conventional physicians are doing the best they can within the system as it stands. As was the case with me, most are simply unaware there could be any other way to approach their profession. The real issue isn't with the doctors, it's that our entire system is set up to *profit from illness.*

Illness Has a Bottom Line

The main difference between holistic and conventional practitioners is that the former are experts in *health* and the latter are experts in *disease.* My personal income dropped by four-fifths when I began practicing holistic medicine. The lower over-all earning potential has nothing to do with poor management. Most of the cost of care is simply *time*—time spent up front figuring out the true underlying root cause(s) of the complaints, followed by time spent educating the patients on how to solve them. On Thursday Clinic days, the entire clinic staff could see, at most, a grand total of seven patients. With our holistic approach, most patients no longer needed ongoing care after just 6–12 months. And, the same approaches and lifestyle changes that *reversed* their former chronic conditions were just as effective at *preventing* new ones from developing in the future.

When you contrast our Centre's approach with the norm seen in most conventional medical clinics today, the differences are striking. In conventional clinics, there are more patients seeking care than there are physicians with time to see them. In an attempt to meet this demand, patients are typically scheduled at 15–20 minute intervals. Usually, only one problem can be discussed per visit. A brief and hurried exam is performed, diagnostic tests are ordered, a follow-up appointment is booked and the patient is sent off to the pharmacy—often feeling more like a number than a human being.

If there is to be any true progress, we must take our focus off the treatment of disease and place it on the *disease of the system.* Let us ask of the system: Where is the financial incentive for physicians to instruct patients on the principles of Wellness when it would mean they no longer require follow-up care? Where is the financial incentive for the pharmaceutical companies to promote true recovery when it would mean patients no longer need their offerings? Perhaps we could take a lesson from the ancient Chinese health philosophy: Pay your doctor only when you are well.[3] After all, shouldn't *results* be the ultimate criteria in health care?

Results Speak Louder than Convention

As we continued to witness astounding results with our patients at the Lexington Centre, I couldn't wait to share my exciting news with the local medical society's program director. Anticipating at least some degree of resistance, I brought along a list of nationally known experts—physicians with great track records of communicating holistic concepts—whom I believed they would want to invite in to speak. I didn't have a clue what I was getting myself into. Instead of thanking me and sharing my enthusiasm, I was shocked to watch them reject the very idea as heretical.

I know that most men,
including those at ease with problems of the greatest complexity,
can seldom accept even the simplest and most obvious truth
if it be such as would oblige them to admit the falsity of conclusions
which they have delighted in explaining to colleagues,
which they have proudly taught to others,
and which they have woven, thread by thread, into the fabric of their lives.

~ Leo Tolstoy (1828–1910)

After meeting with me, the medical society personnel immediately contacted the American Medical Association (AMA). It turned out my experts were already on their alternative "hit list." That was the beginning and the end of my attempts to share my holistic discoveries with the conventional medical societies. From that time on, the word given out by the organized officials in Kentucky to anyone who would listen was, "Dr. Stoll is a *quack!*" But there was no denying the value of what I'd learned, no denying the results—and no turning back. I went on to become a founding member of the American Holistic Medical Association (AHMA) in 1978 and served for several years on its board of trustees.

As word began to spread about the successes at our Centre, IBM (at that time, the largest employer in Lexington) invited me to teach a sixteen-hour Wellness course at their plant. By the end of the first year, the room could no longer hold all the volunteer students wanting to attend. I was then asked to teach the same course (which I renamed "Stress Management Through Wellness") at Transylvania University. During the seven years that I taught there (1977–1984), it remained their most successful and popular evening course.

Our popularity continued to skyrocket. In the spring of 1981, the Kentucky Academy of Family Practice sponsored us in a booth on holistic medicine called "Physician Heal Thyself." Soon after, *PM Magazine* featured a story about our Centre. Then, in the summer of 1982, the Fayette County Medical Society sponsored twenty-two televised sessions of "Doctor Talk" during the CBS evening news about holistic medicine and our Centre. Meanwhile, I was authoring a number of articles for national publications and had become a medical advisor for a number of college textbooks on health, sexuality and drug abuse.

Before I knew it, I found myself deluged with requests for speaking engagements all across the country. For the next eight years, I gave presentations to local and national, lay and professional organizations about combining alternative approaches with conventional medicine. I was featured in the *New York Times* and *Newsweek*, as well as many syndicated newspapers. The downside to this was, more popular I grew in the eyes of the local community, the more the Kentucky medical licensing board (KMLB) countered me with various offensive tactics.

My Medical License: Harassed and Revoked

Despite my initial negative encounter with the program director of my local medical society, I remained predominantly ignorant of the AMA's pattern of threatening the licenses of physicians who became successful in the public eye with offering alternatives to strictly conventional medicine. That is, until it began happening to me. The reason I was targeted was not personal. The story of harassment I'm about to tell is well known by my holistic colleagues throughout the country, and continues today to a certain extent.[4]

The official harassment began in 1980 when the KMLB questioned my use of chelation therapy for selected patients. Since at that time I still believed they were genuinely looking for the facts, I gave them some fifteen hundred references from world literature demonstrating its safety and effectiveness, and told them I would be happy to discuss it with them after they had looked into the research. They never took me up on that offer, and the chelation issue was dropped.

The following year, the KLMB approached me again—this time, asking why I had employed a chiropractor in my office. I challenged them to present me with any documentation showing that employing a chiropractor was unethical, illegal or in any way against Kentucky medical statutes. That was the end of that one.

Next, I was brought before the board for my then-new practice of adding a serum magnesium test to all my basic patient workups. (This was before I learned about the difference between serum and intracellular magnesium testing.) After being told to wait in a separate room while the KMLB spent more than four hours with the Blue Cross Blue Shield representatives, I presented them with over two hundred articles supporting my position. They passed them around for a few minutes, then decreed that "testing for magnesium is an experimental procedure and will not be covered by insurance." Since the test itself only cost about fifty cents, that's when it finally hit me: The complaints brought by these types of committees had nothing to do with the supposed "issue" at hand.

In addition to such frivolous annoyances designed to waste my time and resources, I was also dealing with complaints from local physicians who saw me as a threat to their reputations. For example, a Lexington doctor became upset after I told a patient of his (who had come to me with Type I diabetes) that she had "rampant free-radical pathology." Although he was an internist who specialized in diabetes, he had never heard of free radicals. Rather than call me to inquire, he made an official complaint to the board. In response, I made a copy of a *Wall Street Journal* article on free-radical pathology (featured just that week) and sent it to the board along with a computer search producing more than fifty other articles. I added a comment that perhaps there was a case to be made against a physician who files an official complaint against another based on not knowing the rudiments of his own specialty. The issue was dropped, and of course today the existence of free radicals is widely known.

The following year, after having been a regular guest on the local University of Kentucky National Public Radio (NPR) station (three times per week for several years), I stated on the air that statistics showed only 11% of coronary bypass surgeries could be justified by any scientific standard. Given my popularity in the community, a cardiac surgeon from the Veterans Administration saw my comment as a tangible threat to his practice and filed an official complaint. He was later listed in the national media among surgeons with the poorest track records. Today, these same coronary bypass statistics are widely known and accepted by nearly everyone except the cardiac surgeons themselves.[5]

Other harassment tactics eventually occurred. For example, one day out of the blue, the manager of the radio station was ordered to take me off the air. At first he refused, since conventional physicians already had four times as many slots and he believed the information I offered was valid. He called me into his office and, in tears, said he was originally told that the medical school would withdraw all of its financial support from the station if he didn't comply. When that proved ineffective, they threatened his pension—after thirty years of running that station and within one year of his retirement. If he refused to take me off the air they would demote him to errand boy status and his retirement would be based on that salary rather than his current management position.

As the years went by, the AMA leaned more toward harassing holistic-minded physicians over trivial (often fictitious) complaints unrelated to the practice of alternatives. That way, we not only had to defend against the specific complaint, but were also put in the impossible situation of trying to prove that the *real* reason we were being targeted was due to the promotion of alternatives. This scenario greatly increased the time and cost of each court appearance.

The harassment game, as I've seen it successfully played repeatedly, is as follows: The licensing board makes an accusation against the physician, who is then forced to cancel all patient appointments, hire a lawyer and appear before the board to officially address the "complaint." Then, after being purposely put off for hours on end, the physician is told, "Sorry, we will be unable to hear your case today." The goal—to wear down the physician on every level until no resources remain, financial or otherwise.

The most successful tyranny
is not the one that uses force to assure uniformity
but the one that removes the awareness of other possibilities,
that makes it seem inconceivable that other ways are viable,
that removes the sense that there is an outside.

~ Alan Bloom (1906–2005)

One after the other, the harassments against me continued. After about ten such frivolous episodes, I finally became so disillusioned that I surrendered to the ongoing battle and stopped seeing patients in June of 1993. Physically, emotionally and financially exhausted, I left the state with the intention of taking a one-year sabbatical, turning my practice over to my son Scott who was in residency at the University of Kentucky. Though discouraged, I was determined to keep my license active if for no other reason than the principle involved.

The KMLB, apparently emboldened by my absence, brought yet one more fictitious complaint for which I would have had to travel all the way from Gurnee, Illinois to face. With no income, I could not reasonably make the trip nor hire a lawyer to be there on my behalf. Based on my not showing up, the board revoked my medical license on November 17, 1994.

Going Public with My Story

With my license officially revoked, I had nothing further to lose in dedicating my life to exposing our monopolistic system to the masses. Called to action, I became an outspoken advocate for change. I created my website, "Ask Dr. Stoll," where I have been answering countless health-related questions at no charge via my online bulletin board for over a decade. In 1996, I wrote and published my first book, *Saving Yourself from the Disease-Care Crisis*. Ten years later, I co-authored *Recapture Your Health* with Jan DeCourtney to provide comprehensive support for those implementing the 3LS of Wellness outlined in Section IV of this book.[6]

Although the health-care climate has been slowly changing for the better over the past few decades, it has come too little, too late for those of us already kicked out of practice. To reverse the damage now would prove far too costly. For example, in my case the AMA would have to admit they were wrong, issue a public apology, restore my license without any further testing and pay me about five million dollars in lost income and punitive damages. I'm not holding my breath on that one.

Only by actually *living* the harassment game firsthand, including having witnessed a number of my peers undergo a similar fate, was I able to truly understand how massive lobbying pressure by the pharmaceutical companies directly influences our government *and* our access to anything outside of the conventional treatment paradigm. Only *then* did I fully realize just how powerful the conventional medical establishment had become in the United States, despite the disease-care crisis caused by its failures.

CHAPTER 3

The Conventional Medical Monopoly

Unless we put medical freedom into the Constitution, the time will come when medicine will organize itself into an undercover dictatorship, to restrict the art of healing to one class of men ...

~ Dr. Benjamin Rush
(Co-signer of the Declaration of Independence, 1746–1813)

Allopathy: Just One of Many "Paths"

Long before conventional medicine became the dominant healing philosophy in the United States, many other popular and successful healing philosophies were already in existence—and thriving. Examples include homeopathy, osteopathy, naturopathy, chiropractic, anthroposophical medicine, ayurvedic medicine and traditional Chinese medicine (TCM), as well as several other less well-known healing philosophies from around the world.

In the early nineteenth century, conventional physicians were known as "allopathic physicians" and the practice of conventional medicine was known as "allopathy." Few people today are familiar with this unusual terminology, which originally served to distinguish conventional medicine from its main competition—the opposing healing philosophy of homeopathy. When allopaths later shifted toward the term "conventional," it not only allowed them to avoid being associated with the other "paths" out there, but to conveniently label them "unconventional" as well.

As detailed in the quote that opens this chapter, despite his atomistic stance, Dr. Benjamin Rush accurately predicted the course the medical establishment would ultimately take in the United States. The fact is, for most citizens today, access to health care is dictated by a list of insurance-approved providers, which in turn is dictated by our powerful, profit-driven conventional medical/pharmaceutical complex. Coverage is typically denied for the types of care that would succeed in the areas where conventional medicine fails—chronic health conditions. In other words, due to a sequence of events that began back in the mid-1800s, our health-care system fits the functional definition of a *conventional medical monopoly*.*[1]

Health Care: A Wake-Up Call

This chapter is designed to provide a much-needed wake-up call for anyone concerned with health and health-care reform. I prefer to present my truths directly for those who are ready to receive them, rather than tiptoe around to avoid offending those who are not. Since the Clinton presidency, most Americans have been aware that health-care reform is a pressing issue in the United States. Yet all plans for "reform" continue to ignore important lessons from past mistakes. If we are to find our way out of this mess, we must first understand how we ended up here. You don't need to be a "conspiracy theorist" to believe something untoward has been going on; you only need the facts.

We will begin with a basic summary of the historical evolution of medical ethics in the United States from the mid-1800s forward; describing how political, social and economic influences have resulted in a system tailored more for the benefit of the medical/pharmaceutical complex than for you, the patient. As you will see, like a snowball grows to giant proportions as it rolls down a steep mountain, our monopolistic system formed and expanded upon itself in ways we were powerless to stop.

First, the Formation of the AMA

In 1847, a private organization called the American Medical Association (AMA) was formed. Its purpose: to provide an avenue for conventional medical doctors to share techniques, research and information with their colleagues. The original goal of the AMA was admirable—to raise the

---

* The health-care system in the United States fits the *functional* definition of a conventional medical monopoly—not to be confused with an absolute monopoly.

current standards of medicine in the best interest of the patients. Unfortunately, this goal eventually shifted more and more toward raising physician income and stifling competition in what was once a free market.[2]

According to political commentator Llewellyn H. Rockwell Jr., "Competition among providers—as with any service in a market economy—leads to rational pricing and maximum consumer choice. But this is exactly what the AMA has always sought to prevent. [It] advanced two seemingly innocent propositions in its early days: that all doctors should have a 'suitable education' and that a 'uniform elevated standard of requirements for the degree of MD should be adopted by all medical schools in the USA'... Part of the AMA's real program, which was openly discussed at its conventions and in the medical journals [was] to secure a government-enforced medical monopoly and high incomes for mainstream doctors."[3]

In 1898, William James, MD, the Harvard-trained physician who has been called the father of American psychology, was among many intelligent voices who saw what was happening and attempted to protect us against a monopolistic system of health care. He testified before the Massachusetts legislature in opposition to a bill that would have outlawed "mental healing" or "mind cures" (using the power of thought to heal the body) by non-MDs. He wisely stated, "If medicine were a finished science, such a bill might be possible. But the whole face of medicine changes unexpectedly from one generation to another, in consequence of widening experience." James deplored the unwillingness of his colleagues to investigate the practices they were so quick to condemn, including homeopathy. Although he sympathized with legitimate attempts to protect the public from quackery, he urged his medical peers to fight "... not for licensure and monopoly (but for) freedom and conciliation."[4]

In the early 1900s, conventional medicine was just beginning to come into its glory with its discoveries of anesthesia and the germ theory of disease. These valuable advances made complicated surgical procedures possible for the first time. Meanwhile, pharmaceutical companies had just discovered how to extract the most active essences from herbs, making standardized dosing possible. These impressive new discoveries had the advantage of being proven valid through the laboratory methods of that time. The problem is, it was subsequently suggested that anything that could not be proven *in that way* should no longer be funded by the government. This hasty conclusion, seemingly logical at the time, formed the basis for the way medicine would be approached from that point forward. By the time that logic proved flawed, there was far too much at stake to turn back.

Next, the Flexner Report

Between 1880 and 1903, the number of medical schools (both conventional and alternative) operating in the United States had almost doubled, rising from 90 to 154 schools. The AMA found itself increasingly threatened by its mounting competition. As reported in the *Journal of the American Medical Association (JAMA)* in 1901, "The growth of the profession must be stemmed if individual members are to find the practice of medicine a lucrative profession." For the sake of self-preservation, the AMA created the Council on Medical Education in 1904, and the events leading up to our current monopoly began their downward spiral.

The Council set out to rate all existing medical schools into a class of either A, B or C, with the sole intention of shutting over half of them down (the non-conventional half). To better promote their agenda, the Council purposely delayed publication of their findings until they had secured the approval and backing of the newly formed Carnegie Foundation for the Advancement of Teaching.[5]

During the initial phase, only about three dozen schools were successfully shut down. The AMA's next step was to hire Abraham Flexner (a non-medically trained man who happened to be the brother of the director of the wealthy Rockefeller Institute for Medical Research) to lead the undertaking on behalf of the Carnegie Foundation. Flexner visited the remaining medical schools with the Council's previous findings in hand for comparison, claiming to have thoroughly investigated 69 schools in just 90 days. Doing exactly what the AMA had hired him to do, he wrote the infamous Flexner Report of 1910.[6]

Finally, the Monopoly Takes Hold

The Flexner Report dictated the standards and curriculum for medical schools in the United States, all of which were incompatible with anything outside the conventional approach. Then, congressional action, foolishly taken in response to that biased report, delegated the classification and approval of medical schools to the AMA—giving them *sole power*. The repercussions were enormous. All non AMA-approved schools were shut down, and lavish grants were awarded to the remaining schools from the Rockefeller Foundation. State medical boards (now *also* controlled by the AMA) ruled that doctors must graduate and obtain licensure from an AMA-approved (Class A) school in order to legally practice medicine.

The unfortunate result of giving the AMA this much power was that any approach to medical care except allopathic medicine became virtually outlawed. The AMA further suggested that if we simply stopped wasting our time and resources thinking holistically, we would progress much faster to the ultimate truths. What a monumental error of judgment that was! The conventional medical monopoly and its resulting disease-care crisis is the price we've been paying ever since.[7]

In the 1950s, the doors of the last U.S. homeopathic medical school were effectively closed. It would be thirty years before advances in knowledge and technology, including molecular science, would begin to unravel the mysteries of homeopathic mechanisms and validate some of its scientific principles in the laboratory—let alone the basic mechanical and physiological principles of chiropractic, osteopathic and nutritional medicine. By the time scientists mastered that technology, it was already too late.

Chiropractic doctors fought back, spending ten years and about seven million dollars in legal fees to force the allopathic monopoly to stop officially excluding them from the U.S. health-care system. According to Ken Adachi, "[T]he AMA was found guilty of conspiracy against chiropractors in 1987 by a federal judge and fined a couple million dollars."[8] Once this case went public, allopathic resistance to chiropractic medicine slowly switched from *overt* (out in the open) to *covert* (hidden or secret). Despite the ruling, most health insurance companies *still* refuse to offer coverage for chiropractic care.

Today, a full century after the Flexner Report, conventional medicine stands among the most powerful functional monopolies of all time, costing the public untold amounts of money. Being the only approach that focuses solely on the treatment of disease, it is also the most lucrative. The conventional medical establishment spends more money lobbying our legislators than what all the other healing philosophies combined could possibly muster up to do the same. As stated by the Institute for Health Freedom, "The medical monopoly goes against the capitalist grain of free, unrestricted, non-monopolistic competition in the marketplace."[9] Being that this is a *medical* monopoly, it is also costing lives—and quality of life—the value of which can never truly be measured.

How (and *Why*) the Monopoly Perpetuates Itself

So many deeply ingrained factors are perpetuating the allopathic monopoly today, many of my holistically oriented colleagues despair of it ever changing. A 2003 report entitled "Death by Medicine" states: "... [M]edicine is in need of complete and total reform: from the curriculum in medical schools to protecting patients from excessive medical intervention ... We are fully aware that what stand in the way of change are powerful pharmaceutical companies, medical technology companies and special interest groups with enormous vested interests in the business of medicine. They fund medical research, support medical schools and hospitals and advertise in medical journals. With deep pockets they entice scientists and academics to support their efforts."[10]

Our lives begin to end
the day we become silent about things that matter.

— Martin Luther King, Jr. (1929–1968)

All monopolies, once established, tend to take on a life of their own. The conventional medical monopoly has perpetuated itself for reasons that have very little to do with quality of care. Again, I want to emphasize that conventional medicine itself is an extremely valuable healing philosophy capable of providing *incredible* benefits to humankind. The physicians themselves are not to blame; most of whom have never been exposed to the historical information presented in this chapter. The issue lies in the fact that many of our citizens are being denied both information about—and equal (insurance-covered) access to—the world's many healing philosophies proven effective in the areas in which conventional medicine continually fails.

The medical monopoly exhibits a great deal of psychological control; not only over the way its own graduates think, but over the way the *public* thinks as well. For example, consider the food processing industry. Having been born and raised on a farm, I know there is far more money to be made in the processing of food than in the creating of it. The financial well-being of the food industry is heavily dependent upon a collective belief that food processing is safe, and that refined, preserved, pasteurized, "fortified" and packaged foods are good for you—or at the very least, not injurious to health.

The chemical industry also plays a huge role in this equation. Erosion due to chemical farming techniques has reduced our topsoil from an average of 9.0 inches in 1976 to an average of 5.9 inches in 1995. With this rapid rate of erosion, the United States (presently the world's top food exporter) may be reduced to importing food just to feed itself in the decades to come.[11] The only way to slow soil erosion is organic farming—a very real and present threat to the chemical industry. In the name of self-preservation, research demonstrating the superiority of organic farming must be ridiculed or downplayed, the public must be led to believe that organic produce is a waste of money, and Congress must be heavily lobbied to maintain the status quo of industrialized, geneticized, chemicalized, pesticized "modern" farming and food processing.[12]

Another perpetuator of our monopolistic system is our nation's health insurance industry. Fathom this: The sicker the insured population is, the wealthier the health insurance companies will be. In other words, the more money insurance companies pay out, the more money they make. How can this be? Government regulations permit only a certain profit margin. Once an insurance company's records reflected that health-care costs were going down (people were becoming healthier), they would be forced to reduce their premiums. This, in turn, would force them to start downsizing, laying off employees, selling buildings and so forth. If health insurance companies started offering equal coverage for holistic solutions, the population would be free to choose that which brings the best results. But until or unless we change the *system*, promoting Wellness would be practically suicidal to the health insurance industry.

Since conventional medicine is ineffective at permanently resolving about 85% of all health complaints seen today, is it any wonder the resistance of the establishment is so strong? Just imagine what would become of the most obvious beneficiary of our current monopoly: the pharmaceutical industry!

Big Pharma: Friend or Foe?

Simple logic tells us that the more diseased the population, the more money there is to be made selling prescription and non-prescription drugs. With so little public awareness of (and faith in) alternatives to conventional medicine, the chronic illness created by our system's lack of a Wellness philosophy has created a huge demand for pharmaceuticals. Most physician's waiting and exam rooms are full of posters and give-aways supplied by their local pharmaceutical representatives, whose full-time jobs are to offer attractive incentives to doctors willing to promote and prescribe their products.

If that weren't intrusive enough, none of us can escape the rampant prescription drug advertisements on television, in magazines and on the Internet. Big Pharma repeatedly says, "Ask your doctor" about the latest featured drug. Notice how there's no mention whatsoever that such drugs are almost never designed for (or even capable of) curing what ails you. This advertising practice, known as direct-to-consumer marketing, was actually *illegal* prior to the mid-1980s. In fact, the only two industrialized countries on this planet who have legalized this practice are the United States and New Zealand.[13]

Only an *unaware* public can be hypnotized by these clever ads into believing that the featured drug treatments will result not only in abundant health and energy, but also attractive youthful bodies, perfect relationships, well-behaved children and joyful laughter amidst frolics through green pastures and sunshine! The subliminal messages of such advertisements, when seen through awakened eyes, become truly laughable. Yet there's nothing funny about U.S. citizens being economically forced to try to solve every type of health complaint with one incomplete healing philosophy. This is what I call "trying to force the health-care camel through the eye of the allopathic needle."

Medical research itself is geared toward producing treatments that can be *patented*—the main reason behind why prescriptions are so expensive. Health promotion and disease prevention approaches, on the other hand, could never be patented, so little if any funding is available for conducting studies that would easily prove their safety and effectiveness. No funding, no interest. As long as the pharmaceutical industry continues to call all the shots, the focus of medical research will continue to revolve around more and more treatment-based therapies instead of educating the public on how to prevent disease from occurring in the first place.[14]

Given that all hard-working citizens (including conventional physicians, health insurance agents and pharmaceutical representatives) simply want to earn a decent living, any serious health-care reform *must* create conditions that allow them to do so by promoting Wellness instead of perpetuating illness. As long as conventional medical schools continue to condition students the way I was originally conditioned, such progress will continue to be slow.

Confessions of a Med School Graduate

Despite *overwhelming* evidence of the safety and effectiveness of the world's many natural, low-cost holistic approaches to healing, my colleagues and I received little or no training about them in medical school. We weren't even trained on the basics of nutrition. It would take years before I'd even *begin* to notice the blatant exclusion, let alone understand the history behind it. At best, alternative approaches have been ridiculed or simply ignored. At worst (as with my license revocation), they have been vehemently opposed.[15]

I would summarize the underlying consensus with which I and my fellow medical school students emerged from our training as follows: *The conventional medical approach to disease is the only safe, rational option for intelligent, scientific-minded people in the modern-day world. Any alternatives (including nutritional supplements) are to be viewed with great suspicion as unregulated, unscientific, ineffective and/or downright dangerous.* Today, many similarly trained physicians are just beginning to learn that nothing could be further from the truth.

> ***College isn't the place to go for ideas.***
>
> ~ Helen Keller (1880–1968)

As was the case with me, most conventional physicians truly want to help their patients and have no idea that their minds are shackled by our monopolistic system of disease care. I know from personal experience that when bias against alternative approaches is deeply ingrained during medical school, rarely does it ever occur to the graduating physician that there may, indeed, be good reason to question it. Given the way the entire system is set up, it is extremely difficult—for both conventional physicians and the public—to recognize the *need* for change.

The Flat Earth Mentality

As nineteenth century German philosopher Arthur Schopenhauer once pointed out, every revolutionary advance in recorded history was first preceded by a long period of resistance, ridicule and objection. Only after much agony does any new major philosophy finally become accepted by the mainstream as being obvious all along. Our views on medicine, health and the human body are no exception. As I often say, "'Tis the bonds of which we are unaware that are the most binding of them all." Until or unless we begin to understand that we are bound, we will not even recognize a need to start looking for the ropes.

When I was in practice, the only conventional physicians considering alternative healing approaches were those whose interest was sparked through personal necessity—typically a health crisis of their own or that of a loved one. Once impressed enough to begin rethinking how they'd been doing business, they often found themselves encountering numerous road blocks, including being driven from practice via their state medical licensing boards. I've seen many well-documented threats create a very legitimate fear factor, resulting in physicians who would use a variety of alternatives on themselves and their families, but were afraid to offer or even *mention* them to their own patients.[16] As more and more people are exposed to the invisible limits imposed upon their thinking, it is my hope that such fears will soon be a thing of the past.

When we look at the startling increases in the variety, number and severity of chronic health conditions in the U.S. population at large, the limitations of using *only* the conventional approach become painfully obvious. The question is no longer *what* needs to be done, but *how* to accomplish it. Given conventional medicine's miserable failure in solving our nation's chronic health conditions, we must insist on equal access—and equal insurance coverage—to the many healing philosophies that *do* solve them, whether they make money for the system or not.

Opening the Door to Change

In the late 1980s, there was a movement in California to pass a bill requiring that a treatment had to *work* before an insurance company would be required to pay for it. If only *that* were the law of the land, complementary medicine would be accepted overnight. One small step in that direction occurred in 1992, despite adamant opposition by the AMA (the most financially powerful lobby in this country). Congress established the Office of Alternative Medicine at the National Institutes of Health (NIH). Today, that department is known as the National Center for Complementary and Alternative Medicine (NCCAM). Finally, the United States has an organization dedicated to conducting scientific research in these areas and disseminating its information to the public. Originally, funding for this department was only $2 million per year but today exceeds $100 million per year.

The trend in the U.S. over the last twenty years has also shown that educated people are willing to pay out of pocket for what really works rather than continue to go through their insurance for what doesn't work or is harmful. The January 1993 issue of *The New England Journal of Medicine* reported that in 1990 there were more visits to non-conventional health practitioners than conventional. The fact that none of these holistic visits were covered by insurance proves that people are beginning to vote with their dollars.[17] Additionally, the majority of patients who visited non-conventional health practitioners were of the upper educational and socio-economic strata of the population, dispelling any myth that alternative doctors prey on an ignorant and gullible public.

Radical change is, indeed, possible. In 1995, the government of Australia, whose attitude used to resemble our own, underwent a complete reversal of its approach to health care after a comprehensive analysis proved that patients who availed themselves of complementary approaches spent a lot less of the system's money and were a lot healthier than patients who depended on allopathic approaches alone. Based on that analysis, Australia now encourages the inclusion of all complementary approaches in its health-care system.[18]

Many United States citizens have been speaking out in support of adopting a paradigm similar to that of Australia. By the year 2000, the residents of at least fifteen states, including Arizona, Nevada, North Carolina, West Virginia, Alaska, New York and Florida, rose up to defend their rights to choose alternative and complementary medical approaches. Arizona enjoys an enlightened licensing system for physicians, with a *separate-but-equal* licensing board to protect complementary practitioners. Perhaps if I had gone there to practice when they invited me in 1990, I would still have my license. Then again, I may never have started my website or written my books.

Never doubt that
a small group of thoughtful citizens can change the world.
Indeed, it is the only thing that ever has.

~ Margaret Mead (1901–1978)

As of this book's printing, attempts at "health-care reform" are still focused on health-care *insurance* reform. Until or unless reform efforts begin to focus on prevention and a Wellness lifestyle, true progress will not be possible. The seeds of destruction of any faulty system lie within it. I believe the present system will eventually collapse under its own weight, coming to an inevitable head of greed and corruption much like the 2008 economic crash. Both share similar patterns: lucrative profits for the elite few at the expense of the majority, unethical and secretive practices, influence over public opinion and a strong resistance to change no matter what the cost.

As we move forward into the next decade and beyond, the question we need to ask ourselves is this: What would happen to the current high cost of health care, and to our individual health profiles, if our system could be set up to profit from Wellness rather than illness?

CHAPTER 4

Beyond Disease Care

Men occasionally stumble over the truth,
but most of them pick themselves up
and hurry off as if nothing has happened.

~ Sir Winston Churchill
(Prime minister of the UK, 1874–1965)

Conventional Medicine *Is* Valuable!

Despite the harm often caused by our country's insistence that we try to solve every type of health complaint with one solitary and incomplete healing philosophy, there's no denying that conventional medicine is *extremely* valuable in and of itself, and is in fact the *only* approach that works for certain medical conditions. It's the conventional medical *system*, not the healing philosophy itself, that is the problem.

One of conventional medicine's recent outstanding achievements was the mapping of the human genome. The Human Genome Project (1990–2000) was a joint venture between the U.S. Department of Energy and the National Institutes of Health. They not only identified all the genes present in human DNA, their findings also validated the fact that only 10–20% of our health conditions are caused by defects in the genome.[1] In other words, the results have proven that more often than not, it's environmental conditions and lifestyle—not genetics—that determines the expression of health or dis-ease.

All the world's various healing philosophies have value, and conventional medicine is no exception. Given the information presented thus far in this book, you may be asking yourself: "How do I determine which healing philosophy (or combination thereof) is best for my unique health concerns?"

The answer to that question must take into account the previously given foundational understanding of the difference between *acute* and *chronic* health conditions as well the difference between a *treatment* and a *cure*.

However, to be more specific and with some notable exceptions, conventional medicine would be my first choice for surgery (when truly necessary, many are not); certain acute bacterial infections; structural congenital conditions; blockage of drainage by stones (kidney, gallbladder and salivary glands); emergencies like appendicitis, acute poisoning, broken bones, lacerations and serious trauma; life support techniques for rare, self-limited conditions like Guillain-Barré syndrome or polio; and certain types of cancer, such as basal cell carcinoma, testicular cancer or Hodgkin's lymphoma (not an all-inclusive list).

The important distinction here is that the aforementioned are all *acute* health conditions. *Chronic* health conditions, on the other hand, are much better managed by the various "unconventional" healing philosophies being denied equal access in this country. Our bodyminds are extremely complex. If we truly want to learn how to prevent and reverse today's most common chronic and degenerative conditions, we must be willing to back up and look at the bigger picture of health and dis-ease. We can begin by acknowledging that there are many different ways any one individual's bodymind might react to the very same underlying causes.

Biochemical Individuality

The various manifestations of all the chronic health conditions in Section III of this book are simply examples of our biochemical individuality. In fact, no two people are biologically identical. Considering that every person has a unique face and physical features, imagine how much more complex and diverse our inner physiology must be. Such biochemical individuality was recognized and described years ago by professor Dr. Roger Williams, who first began publishing his ideas in the 1950s. Through genetic research and gene mapping, we now have proof of what he was talking about. Dr. Williams was a pioneer in nutrition and biochemistry and author of over twenty books and three hundred articles.[2]

As an example of our biochemical individuality, consider this: Genetic research has thus far established at least 40,000 different "inborn errors of metabolism" (essentially, metabolic birth defects), and more are being discovered each month.[3] These defects (differences) often cause *profound* alterations in the way each individual responds to the same environmental stressors or stimuli.

Our biochemical individuality also explains why a particular medication works well for one individual and not for another, and why one person ends up with arthritis, depression or chronic fatigue (for example) whereas another person may end up with diabetes, heart disease or chronic acne—*from the very same causes.* One of the great aspirations of conventional medicine is to correct these inborn errors of metabolism by inserting what is missing back into the defective gene via a viral carrier. It is only a matter of time before we will succeed in that endeavor.

Eventually, the Human Genome Project will open even more doors for conventional medicine to do amazing things other healing modalities cannot, such as stem cell therapy and changing structural congenital abnormalities (both macro and molecular) in utero and thereafter. These and other valuable advances seemed more like science fiction than reality only a few decades ago.

There is no denying the many effective, cutting-edge and life-saving conventional medical treatments available today. Yet when it comes to preventing and reversing the *chronic* health conditions so prevalent in modern society, conventional medicine is at a loss. For these, only proper education—followed by action—will suffice. We must take steps toward improving health rather than viewing our symptoms as annoyances that can be quick-fixed so we can get on with our busy lives.

Symptoms: Messages from the Bodymind

When you are suffering, there's nothing inherently "wrong" with taking advantage of one or more of the available symptom-suppressing treatments for short-term relief. However, if you do not at the same time work toward discovering—and reversing—the underlying root causes (the *why*) of your symptoms, you are playing a potentially dangerous game. If the prescription treatment works well, you may mistakenly believe your problem has been solved. On the contrary, nothing could be further from the truth!

Treating symptoms without addressing the cause is like cutting the wires to your doorbell so you can't hear your neighbor trying to warn you that your house is on fire, or putting tape over the warning lights on the dashboard of your car so you can pretend your engine doesn't need immediate attention. When you short-circuit the messages your bodymind is trying to send you, rest assured it will eventually shout louder—in the form of a new, more serious condition.

Unfortunately, the willingness to *do what it takes* to change is often directly proportional to the degree of suffering currently being faced. Patients who refuse to take the responsibility for their own health off their doctor's shoulders tend to live their lives recklessly and then claim to be victims of their mysterious illnesses. Some people have to "hit bottom" before that willingness will appear, which in many cases could be diabetes, terminal cancer or an autoimmune disease.

The individuals least likely to change are those who mock the very things and people that would improve their health and quality of life. Health is a choice, and like all worthwhile things, it takes effort. People who aren't willing to put forth the effort will go to great lengths to avoid the emotional pain of admitting their own role in their misery. They blame their poor health on bad luck, bad genes, bad doctors or the characteristics of their particular diagnosis—*anything* but their own lifestyle choices.

Our bodies communicate to us clearly and specifically, if we are willing to listen to them.

~ Shakti Gawain (born 1948)

Persistent symptoms don't occur without reason. Think of your symptoms as messages from your bodymind that you can't afford to ignore. The problem with ignoring the mild symptoms, signals and alerts your bodymind is trying to send you is that you are likely to eventually learn about more serious messages firsthand. In other words, your bodymind tends to shout *louder* if you don't heed the earlier messages.

Pill Popping: The *Whoops!* Factor

Wise healers throughout the ages have said the same thing: "Illness is an opportunity for learning." Many people would rather pop pills and remain in denial than do what it takes to implement the necessary changes into their lifestyle to be well. In all seriousness, I've seen people die of cancer, heart attacks or strokes because of their unwillingness to change. Simply reading and learning about what must be done is only the first step. *Doing what it takes* to solve your chronic conditions takes commitment, effort and persistence.

In my experience, the most efficient and least painful path back to health lies in combining the best of all healing philosophies. While enjoying symptomatic relief from your conventional treatment(s), use this time as a window of opportunity to reverse the underlying causes of your dis-ease. This book will illustrate the way. Armed with the proper information, you have one of two choices: long-term dependence on your doctor and your drugs, or doing what it takes to achieve abundant health so you eventually no longer need either.

In an ideal world, the decision to undergo treatment is a mutual one between a doctor and his or her well-informed patient. But in reality, few people bother to do their own research. If your only source of medical education is what you are getting during your 15-minute office visits, you may never be aware that drugs are prescribed on a trial-and-error basis. You may also never understand that the potential benefits of any treatment must be weighed against potential risks, many of which are unknown.

Many of our nation's elderly are taking so many prescribed drugs, they end up needing additional prescriptions just to treat the side effects. They're essentially trading one condition for two or three new ones. Even worse, they may be visiting multiple doctors and specialists, many of whom are unaware of the medications being prescribed by the others. Have you ever stopped to wonder what "side effects" are, if not new dis-eases?

It is easy to get a thousand prescriptions
but hard to get one single remedy.

~ Chinese Proverb

Even when only *one* prescription is taken, since every individual's biochemistry is unique, there's no way to accurately predict the long-term effects of any particular medication—especially in developing children. Not only may a drug prove ineffective, it may also cause unanticipated and irreversible harm. Sometimes it takes twenty years or more for the "Whoops! factor" to rear its ugly head, which is why so many law firms specialize in suits related to prescription drugs.

What You Don't Know *Can* Hurt You

Few people are aware of the facts being presented in this book, let alone the potential risks of blindly following a "make it all go away" approach. If you were to conduct a survey on the street and ask, "What are the three leading causes of death in the United States?" most would never name "conventional medicine" as one of the three. Yet in the year 2000, conventional medical treatments were the third leading cause of death, behind heart disease and cancer. More recent statistics have moved this figure to number *one*. A 2003 National Vital Statistics report concluded, "It is evident that the American medical system is the leading cause of death and injury in the United States.[4]

"First, do no harm," indeed!

Conventional physicians have been trained to look at dis-ease by focusing intently on each individual symptom as if it existed independent of the bodymind system as a whole. That approach may be effective for many acute health conditions (about 15% of those seen in family practice clinics), but is a complete disaster as a solution to *chronic* health conditions (about 85% of those seen). Chronic health conditions are caused by a combination of factors, all of which are described in the first two sections of this book. When these factors finally come together to overwhelm the body's natural ability to defend and repair itself, chronic dis-ease is the result. Conventional medicine admits—but rarely advertises—that it doesn't even have very good *treatments* for chronic health conditions, let alone *cures*.

As a physician, I can assure you that most conventional doctors are often given way too much credit when it comes to the extent of their knowledge and expertise. Some don't bother to keep up with research in their own field, let alone the latest in holistic philosophies. When I graduated from medical school, as long as we passed the exam, our board certifications were issued with no expiration dates.[5] In other words, we never had to crack open another book or keep up with the latest in medical research from that day forward!

Since 1970, new board certifications began carrying a 6–10 year expiration date. Although this is an improvement, board certification is optional and is completely separate from being "licensed." In other words, once licensed a physician can continue to practice medicine with or without that board certification. Since the statistics on death and injury from medical intervention is so high, in one sense you could say doctors have a "license to kill." Ignorance is *not* bliss. If illnesses were truly caused by a deficiency of the drugs used to treat them, we would be the healthiest nation on the planet!

Let Those Who Have Ears, Hear

The long-term cure for chronic health conditions will never be found in a bottle. Think of it this way: If you mow over a large weed in the middle of your grass, it may become unnoticeable for a few days. But rest assured, as long as the root remains intact, it will return. Eventually, it will also create new weeds.

Thankfully, some of the most blatantly obvious lifestyle-disease connections (such as diet and its role in obesity-related dis-eases) are finally being acknowledged by the media and brought to the forefront. During the first fifteen years of my practice, my colleagues and I feared offending and alienating our patients by even *suggesting* that their day-to-day lifestyle choices just *might* have something to do with their illnesses. Even today, not every patient is ready and/or willing to hear that their own habits are dramatically increasing or decreasing the length and quality of their lives, dramatically increasing or decreasing their resistance to illness, as well as reversing or accelerating the progression of chronic disease and/or aging.

Illness has a bottom line. There is a *lot* of money to be made treating symptoms! Might it follow that the system making all that money would be very reluctant to fund research on lifestyle and preventive techniques? Nutrition, exercise and relaxation cannot be patented. These and other "home remedies" are still considered by the AMA as competition. If there were fortunes to be found in promoting a Wellness lifestyle, most chronic health conditions would have been solved and prevented long ago.

Moving *Beyond Disease Care*

To protect yourself from becoming a statistic, the first goal ought to be the prevention of dis-ease via the promotion of Wellness. Then, if you do happen to become ill or symptomatic, the next goal would be two-fold: safe and effective treatments to relieve suffering in the short term, along with lifestyle changes to remove the factors that potentially created the condition in the first place. The problem is that most people only pursue the treatment half of the equation.

Every single cell is a perfect microcosm of the entire human being. The natural tendency of all life is to follow the path of least resistance. That means, humans are unlikely to change their ways until or unless enough of their bodies' cells shout for attention (a measure of how sick they are). Likewise, every single human is a perfect microcosm of the entire human species. Until enough people in this country shout loud enough to demand change in the *system*, the system is unlikely to change *its* ways.

The next section of the book will detail the processes by which chronic health conditions come into being, including the role of "stress" and the environment. The Serenity Prayer states: "God, grant me the serenity to accept the things I cannot change, the courage to change the things I can, and the wisdom to know the difference."[6] We may not be able to change our genetics (as of yet), nor do we have the power to change many aspects of the environment. But we are *far* from powerless when it comes to changing our habits of lifestyle.

No matter what your current status of health, decide what steps you are willing to take toward recovery. Some people jump in and do a 180-degree turnaround; others do better by picking just one or two things to change at a time. If you made one specific lifestyle change every 2–4 weeks, imagine the health improvements you'll be enjoying a year from now! After reading this book cover to cover, create a plan you can live with and *stick to it*. The noticeable improvements in your health will motivate you to take the next step, and the next …

Section II

PRECURSORS TO CHRONIC HEALTH CONDITIONS

The Eye-Opening Truth
about *Stress*

CHAPTER 5

Modern Medical Interpretation of Stress

Formerly, when religion was strong and science weak,
men mistook magic for medicine;
now, when science is strong and religion weak,
men mistake medicine for magic.

~ Thomas Szasz
(Humanist of the Year, 1973)

Stress: It's *Not* Just Your Daily Frustrations

What comes to mind when you hear the word "stress"? Do you associate it with things like living in a demanding and fast-paced society, traffic jams, conflicts with the boss, problems with the neighbors, marital discord, rebellious children and financial strain? People talk every day about the major and minor events in their lives that are causing them to feel "stressed out." It seems the word "stress" has become an accepted catch-all term for anything frustrating, exhausting or emotionally upsetting. But what is stress, *really*?

There is no doubt the above examples do belong under the "stress" umbrella. However, these psychosocial (psychological plus social) stressors comprise only a small fraction (about 10%) of the total number we humans experience on a daily basis. The remaining 90% are actually derived from a variety of physical and environmental sources: electromagnetic, atmospheric, nutritional, hormonal, chemical, bacterial and viral (*not* an all-inclusive list).[1]

You may have seen those little quizzes in books and magazines for ranking the stress impact of various life events. The quiz assigns point values for stressful events experienced within the past 1–2 years, such as marriage, divorce, loss of a job, change in career, change in residence, birth of a child, death of a loved one, diagnosis of a disease and so forth (perpetuating the fiction in the public's mind that "stress" is purely psychosocial). Your total score is supposed to predict the likelihood of your experiencing a stress-related illness in the near future. Talk about a self-fulfilling prophecy! Given that quantum mechanics has shown our thoughts, beliefs, observations and expectations create and influence our experience of reality, such a prediction is potentially *dangerous.*[2]

Back in 1977, I thought I had a professional understanding of what stress was. After all, I had been practicing medicine for fourteen years and teaching medical school for four years. I had a degree in psychology and a keen interest in the effect of the mind on the body. Yet despite all of that, it wasn't until a patient of mine gave me the book, *Mind as Healer, Mind as Slayer* by Kenneth Pelletier, MD that my eyes really began to open to a much broader understanding on the topic of stress.[3]

Though written back in 1978, I still consider Dr. Pelletier's book the best introduction I've ever read as far as a practical *medical* understanding of the effects of chronic stress on human physiology. Neurosurgeon C. Norman Shealy, MD, PhD stated on the cover, "America's medical expenses could be cut in half if everyone put in practice the principles outlined in Dr. Pelletier's book. I highly recommend it." Little did I know that within a year of reading this book, I would be joining Dr. Shealy as a founding member of the American Holistic Medical Association (AHMA).

Back in 1926, the father of the modern theory of stress, Hans Selye, MD, came up with three definitions for "stress:" 1) the nonspecific response of the body to any demand, 2) the rate of wear and tear within the body, and 3) the state manifested by a specific syndrome consisting of all the non-specifically induced changes within a biological system. Selye also came up with his now-famous theory to describe the influence of stress on dis-ease, a phenomenon which he termed the General Adaptation Syndrome (G.A.S.). The G.A.S. is defined as: "the manifestations of stress in the whole body, as they develop over time."[4]

Stress, then, is basically *anything that requires the body to adapt.* This chapter will demonstrate the exact mechanisms behind how all stressors affect health—both directly and indirectly.

Environmental Stressors: 90% of the Load

Take a moment to ponder what life was like just two hundred years ago, before things such as electricity, radio broadcasting, telephone lines, automobiles, computers, microwaves, cell phones, video games, pesticides, herbicides, high-tech food manufacturing and preservatives entered the picture. Then, ponder how few of these frequencies and substances can be perceived with your five physical senses. Regardless of your inability to see, hear, taste, touch or smell most of them, *all* environmental stressors have a constant and cumulative effect on your bodymind.

Sources of Environmental Stressors[5]

- **Electromagnetic (EMF)**: Examples include power lines, radio waves, mobile phones, televisions, computers, electrical appliances, baby monitors, microwaves, x-rays and radar.
- **Chemical:** Examples include pesticides, herbicides and toxic cleaning products in the form of vapors, gasses, mists, fumes and dust—both inhaled and absorbed through the skin.[6]
- **Physical:** Examples include noise, vibration, extremes of temperature and improper illumination.
- **Biological:** Examples include mold, fungi, bacteria and insects.
- **Nutritional:** Examples include improper diet and trace nutrient deficiencies due to the food refining process.

A study completed in 1987 reported that the average person in this culture is exposed to over a thousand times more stressors per person per day as compared to just one hundred years earlier. This calculated to an estimate of over 382,000 stressors per person per day, a number that has continued to increase at an alarming rate.[7] Keep in mind that this study came *before* rapid technological advances in security, convenience and entertainment led to electronic gadgets such as mobile (cell) phones and innumerable wireless devices.

The chemical industry is a major player, having created a plethora of environmental stressors, all of which are relatively new to humanity as a species. According to the Alliance for a Clean Environment (ACE), "The chemical manufacturing industry is the single largest industrial source of developmental and neurological toxic emissions (to air and water) in the U.S.... The overwhelming majority of chemicals in use have never been tested for specific effects on the physical and brain development of children. More than half (53%) of all toxic chemical releases reported to the federal Toxins Release Inventory are known or suspected developmental toxins or neurotoxins."[8] No wonder our alternative medicine practitioners are trying so hard to educate their patients about the necessity of detoxification and cleansing diets.

The only good is knowledge and the only evil is ignorance.

~ Socrates (470–399 BC)

Further adding to the problem, 80% of the prepared foods we now consume contain genomically altered substances.[9] We've yet to discover the short and long-term effects these "frankenfoods" (genetically modified or "GM" foods) may be having on the population—especially our children. One telling clue might be the fact that the dramatic increase in peanut allergy began with genetically modified peanuts.[10] As of this printing, there are *still* no laws protecting our right to know whether the foods we are buying, eating and serving to our children have been genetically altered.

The suspected harmful effects of cell phones and cell phone towers may soon prove more devastating than anyone could have predicted. The frequent use of cell phones is now widely believed to be the number one cause of the recent increase in brain tumors, especially in children.[11] Because we Americans love our conveniences so much, it's no surprise we don't want to see, hear or believe the mounting evidence and dire predictions about the effects these current and future exposure rates might have on the long-term health of ourselves, our children and our planet.

Electromagnetic Soup

Electromagnetic frequencies (EMFs) produced by our technologically advanced way of life make up the fastest growing category of stressors. Medical researchers at the turn of the 19th century tried to tell us that the body is an electromagnetic machine at least as much as it is a structural and chemical machine, but they were laughed off the stage because the technology to prove this theory didn't exist until many decades later. Today, we can observe the effect of even the smallest electrical and magnetic fields on the very atoms and molecules within our cells by using instruments like the SQUID (superconducting quantum interferometer device).[12] These electromagnetic fields can have either a positive or a negative effect on our cells, depending on their *frequency* and *dose*.*

The majority of the EMFs humans have created wreak havoc with our cells and their messages. According to Andrew Weil, MD, "Electromagnetic pollution may be the most significant form of pollution human activity has produced in this century, all the more dangerous because it is invisible and insensible."[13] The extent to which these tiny traces of electromagnetism influence our most basic atomic and molecular metabolism is currently unknown.

Since most Americans can no longer escape EMFs, the best thing to do is make a conscious effort to minimize exposure.** Unplug all electrical devices not in use, and try to keep as much distance as possible between you and your gadgets—such as computer monitors, television screens, microwaves, wireless phones, electric clocks and even light bulbs, especially any electrical devices near and around your bed.[14]

In my estimation, there are now more than 200,000 types of man-made electromagnetic frequencies in our environment, none of which existed in nature just two hundred years ago. It's as if we are being literally

---

* Messages are continually sent back and forth between molecules within our cells. Magnets have been shown to alter their trajectory—thus the science behind magnet therapy.

** To measure the EMF or ambient electricity being generated by the electronic gadgets in your home, you can purchase a simple and relatively inexpensive device called a Gauss meter. When I tested my own home many years ago, I was surprised to find that the device radiating the most intense electromagnetic smog was our video cassette rewinder. This was the case even when it wasn't running, but simply plugged in.

soaked in the "electromagnetic soup" humankind has created. Chances are, we won't be able to ignore their effects on our human physiology for much longer. The following two stories illustrate how a relatively *new* stressor might affect a population.

Power Lines and Radio Waves

In the 1950s, a small, remote village in Switzerland was noted for being practically free of most of the diseases of modern civilization (arthritis, cancer, cardiovascular disease, mental disorders, etc.). In addition, the inhabitants of this village seemed to live very long, productive lives, much like the Hunza people in the former U.S.S.R. Impressed by the villagers' superior health, the Swiss government decided to study the entire community. As an incentive to participate in the study, the government offered to run power lines up the mountains into the village. The villagers, having never had electricity up to that point, agreed and the lines were run.

Within five years, the first signs of disease so common in the rest of the civilized world began to appear. Within twenty years, the incidence of disease in the village was nearly identical to the rest of the country and, for the first time, the average age at death began to fall. Since the addition of new electromagnetic fields was the only discernable factor that had changed, the Swiss government wanted to shut off the power lines immediately. By that time however, the villagers had become so attached to their electrical conveniences they refused to part with their power lines. In fact, they would sooner die than be inconvenienced—not an uncommon attitude in *our* country.

This reminds me of what happened to Guglielmo Marconi in 1896 when he went to the British Isles to set up the first radio broadcasting station. Within a few months of the station's completion, someone tried (and failed) to assassinate him. The interrogated perpetrator said something to this effect: "My family was always completely healthy until you turned on that infernal radio broadcasting station. Now they are always sick, can't sleep and are generally miserable. I'm going to kill the man that did this to us!" Until Marconi's death more than thirty years later, the record number of attempts on his life made it necessary for him to have about fifty bodyguards. The common story of every assailant was the same: "Those radio waves are killing us!"

EMF: An Invisible Burden

Prior to Marconi's first radio broadcasting station, the only electromagnetic frequencies present in the environment were lightning and the Van Allen Belts (magnetic fields around the earth). These natural fields beat at 7.4 cycles per second which is, coincidentally, right in the middle of the brain-wave frequency range that creates the *relaxation response* in the body.

Having been surrounded by electromagnetic frequencies all our lives, most of us have no frame of reference for what it might feel like to actually be free of exposure. One way to find out is to make a chicken-wire Faraday Cage and sit in it for 15–20 minutes. A Faraday Cage is a 360-degree sphere of wire netting which effectively blocks out the usual electromagnetic soup surrounding us on an everyday basis. Once inside, you will have no doubt that some kind of burden has been temporarily lifted. If that doesn't impress you, just wait and see what you notice when you exit the cage.

How to Make a Faraday Cage

1. Purchase chicken wire or fine-mesh metal screening from any building supply or old-fashioned hardware store (copper is recommended, but any conductive material will work). Chicken wire has 1–2 inch hexagonal or octagonal holes and is sold in two and eight-foot wide rolls.
2. Using the chicken wire or mesh, form a hollow cage big enough to sit in (sphere, square or rectangle shaped), fastening the strips together with wire or twist ties. For structural strength, it is fine and even desirable for the strips of wire to overlap when making your cage. Be sure there are no gaps larger than the manufactured holes.
3. Cut an opening big enough for you to easily get in and out of, leaving one side uncut to act as a hinge. Bend over the ends of any sharp wires to avoid injury. You may also want to ground the cage to a copper water pipe with a couple of #6 cables.
4. To test the cage, take a portable radio inside. You should be unable to receive any AM or FM station.

Each individual stressor combines and interacts with every other individual stressor, magnifying the stress-effect of each as well as their individual effects. Since virtually *none* of our current environmental stressors existed just two centuries ago, and since so many new stressors have appeared within just the last few decades, there's no question the increase in chronic health conditions is directly related to the collective burden of today's modern high-tech society. *All* stressors, whether environmental or psychosocial, decrease the body's available reserves for keeping dis-ease at bay.

Reserves: Your Body's Bank Account

Every organ system in your body has a certain ratio of *reserves*. Think of reserves as an extra amount of function or energy stored up for possible future use, much like a bank account. As long as you don't try to withdraw more than you have, all is well. If 95% of your liver was removed, your body could still function normally as long as the remaining 5% was perfectly healthy. However, you could not then "afford" to get hepatitis at that point because your liver wouldn't have enough reserves left to cope with the disease. Likewise, if one and a half of your lungs were removed, you could still run a marathon as long as the remaining half a lung was perfectly healthy.

The same scenario applies to all organ systems in the body—and most importantly, the immune system. If, for example, the average American is forced to use 90% of all available reserves just trying to cope with the overwhelming number of environmental stressors, that leaves only 10% for dealing with life's psychosocial stressors. No wonder emotional crises so often lead to illness and dis-ease. The *form* it takes will vary. Knowing your family medical history can give you an idea as to which illnesses you may be predisposed to genetically ("nature"), so you can focus your attention toward prevention ("nurture"). Keep in mind that genetic predispositions are merely *tendencies*—rarely are they absolutes.

The chronic health conditions covered in Section III of this book are representative examples of how the burden of excessive stress expresses itself according to our individual genetic predispositions. Forewarned is forearmed, but not in the sense we've been conditioned to think. Conventional practitioners look at family history so they can search for early signs of disease (for which they will make billions of dollars treating). Holistic practitioners focus on removing the barriers to health so disease can be prevented and/or reversed.

The Missing Half of the Equation

Consider the standard allopathic medical approach to preventing common illnesses such as colds and flu. Based on the germ theory of disease, almost all efforts have focused on avoiding exposure to the viruses that cause them. Of course, germs *can* and *do* cause illness, but avoidance is only one aspect of a much bigger picture. Despite our best efforts, we will always be *surrounded* by germs—avoiding exposure is impossible!

Remember how Mom always made you bundle up when you went outside in the winter so you wouldn't catch a cold (which would make no sense according to the germ theory of disease)? As it turns out, she was on to something. Of course, it isn't the cold temperatures that *cause* the illness directly. But the ice cold air *can* be the additional stressor that, when the body is already at the limit of its reserves, throws your immune system over the threshold so that it can no longer keep the already present cold virus at bay.

Similarly, consider the swine flu scare of 2009–2010. The media portrayed images of entire communities walking around with masks on their faces. People were terrified of "catching" the disease. The media failed to mention that the difference between those who get sick and those who remain healthy depends a lot more on variations in individual immune system reserves than exposure to germs.

The Bell Curve of Immunity

The "immune system" refers to a complex network of organs, tissues, molecules and cells whose job it is to defend the body against unwanted invaders such as bacteria, viruses, fungi, parasites and cancer. Since the immune system is such an important system in the body, it should come as no surprise that it stores as much as 1,000 times its base requirements in reserves. Still, the immune system, like *all* body systems, has its limits. The amount of reserves available to any given individual at any given time varies widely depending on that person's unique genetic, environmental and lifestyle factors.

If we were to draw a diagram representing the immune capacity of the entire population, we would end up with an inverted U-shape known as a bell curve. At the extreme left of the curve are those born with practically no immune capacity, such as the "bubble boy" who'd be unable to survive if he ventured out of his sterile protective bubble. At the extreme right of the curve are the "lucky ones" who were born with practically infallible immunity, such as the 105-year-old man who, when interviewed about how he managed to live such a long and healthy life replies, "I smoked and drank a lot, ate fast food and ran with wild women. All these 'health nuts' are crazy—what a waste of time!"

Unlike these extreme examples, most of us are born with average immune capacity, as represented by the top center of the curve in the illustration below. Whenever health is discussed relative to the entire population, be careful not to confuse the terms "average" and "normal" with the terms "healthy" or "optimal."

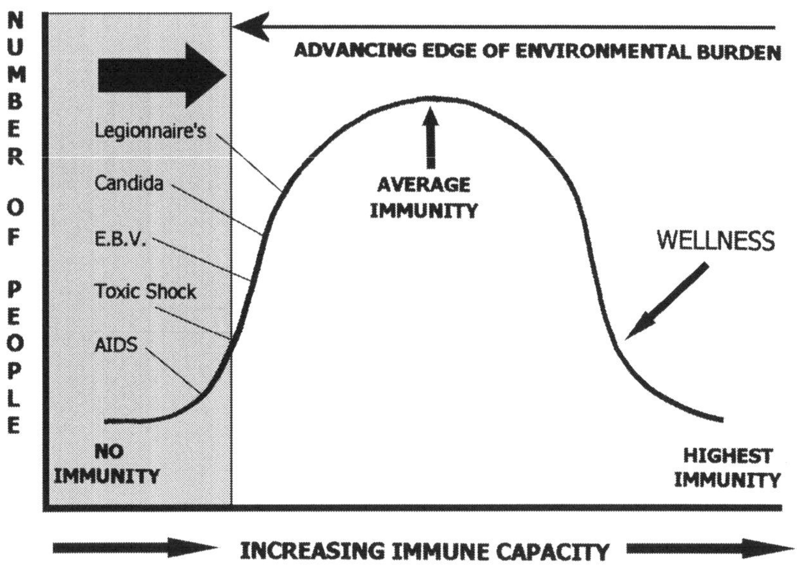

Bell Curve of Immunity

As shown in the graph on the previous page, the "advancing edge of environmental burden" (stress) is gradually overwhelming the percentage of the population who happen to have been born toward the left side of the bell curve. AIDS, multiple chemical sensitivity (MCS) and chronic fatigue syndrome (CFS) are just a few recent examples of a rapidly increasing list of diagnoses that didn't even exist just a few generations ago.[15] Depending on your age, you may remember a time when cancer and AIDS were virtually unheard of. Such "new" diseases always arise *first* in people with compromised immune systems.

Since stress wreaks havoc on our physical, mental, emotional and spiritual well-being, it is accurate to say that most illnesses have a *psychosomatic* component. This is not the same as implying it's "all in your head" or suggesting you are a hypochondriac. The true definition of psychosomatic is, "relating to bodily systems caused by mental or emotional disturbance." In other words, psychosomatic symptoms are *very real* symptoms brought about by chronic stress accumulation. Psychosomatic illnesses and dis-eases are no less real.

Rabies Is a Psychosomatic Disease!

During my years of giving lectures and conducting workshops around the country, I used a study about rabies in rats as a teaching example. This study, done in the 1960s, was inspired by Hans Selye's then recently published work on stress.[16] I started my comments to a group of attendees by declaring, "Rabies is a psychosomatic disease!" This never failed to get the participants' attention since, according to common knowledge, the statement appears to be blatantly false. Obviously, rabies is caused by the rabies virus, right?

The most efficient way to ensure infection for such studies was to inject the live rabies virus directly into the rats' brains. Yet there were always a few rats that baffled the researchers by appearing to be immune to the disease. These resistant rats were simply excluded and forgotten (no surprise to me, since conventional medicine's focus is the study of disease, not health.) However in one particular study, a group of enlightened researchers decided to conduct a study on the rats that stayed healthy after being injected with the virus. Of course, thousands of rats had to die in order to collect enough resistant rats to do the experiment. The researchers then subjected the resistant rats to food deprivation, loud unexpected noises, flashing lights and unusual variations in temperature. In effect, they were *stressed*. These previously healthy rats then all developed rabies and died.

Like a small percentage of humans, these particular rats happened to be born with superior immune systems. They had sufficient innate immune reserves to hold the rabies virus at bay *until* they were stressed beyond capacity. The combination of the burden of holding the rabies virus at bay *plus* the burden of adapting to the new additional stressors finally overwhelmed the rats, allowing the dormant virus to become active.

Without the additional stressors, the rats would have lived until a combination of old age and circumstance eventually lowered their immune reserves, at which point, they would have finally developed rabies and died. This same mechanism explains why a person can develop shingles during a time of great stress, and why many people who are HIV-positive live as long as ten years before coming down with full-blown AIDS (and some *never* develop the illness).

AIDS Research and the Immune System

The AIDS epidemic has been one of those cruel tragedies that contains a valuable message. In one sense, AIDS is a godsend because it represents diseases serious enough to get the attention of the majority of the population. This severe immunological disease is caused by the HIV (human immunodeficiency) virus, transmitted primarily through contaminated body fluids such as blood and semen. The virus specifically and directly targets and attacks the immune cells of the body.

AIDS research has shown that a combination of stress reduction techniques, regular exercise and a natural diet of Whole Foods (the basic tenets of the 3LS), along with high doses of certain vitamins, produced the longest period of time of any therapy yet known, between HIV-positive status and the actual appearance of AIDS.[17] This dispels the theory of an "incubation period," as was commonly discussed among experts in the field. Some HIV-positive individuals live out their normal life spans without *ever* getting full-blown AIDS. Others become ill immediately after testing because the psychological stress of receiving the devastating news pushes their immune system reserves beyond maximum capacity. Like the rats just described, they can no longer keep the virus at bay.[18]

AIDS is just one historic example of a huge variety of what we doctors call the "new disease of the month." All such diseases and epidemics are caused by the same basic mechanisms—depletion of immune reserves. In 1985, I was given the privilege of describing the American Holistic Medical Association's (AHMA) position on AIDS, based on the published literature of that time. As I stated in my speech: "Holistic medicine has known the cause of (and the solution to) AIDS since shortly after the problem was made public. The HIV virus is an opportunist. It can only infect someone whose immunity is already compromised … Obviously, the HIV virus has been around for thousands of years. Why is it causing an epidemic now?"

Today, people are being diagnosed with irritable bowel, cancer, fibromyalgia, Lyme disease and a long list of other chronic conditions unheard of just a century ago. Far too many patients do not yet understand the fact that the allopathic approach cannot "clear up" such diseases with some magical pill. Fortunately, we all have the power to improve our health and our quality of life. We can take actions toward increasing our immune reserves (thus improving our chances of getting or remaining well) and we can consciously avoid things that decrease our immune reserves (thereby reducing our susceptibility to illness). This book will help you do exactly that.

Are You Walking on the Edge?

To better understand how lifestyle plays a role in either increasing or decreasing reserves, I will use the following analogy. Imagine you are leisurely walking down a sidewalk when all of a sudden you trip over a rock. For our analogy, the rock you tripped over would be called the "stressor" and what you felt inside your bodymind (fright and/or perhaps pain) would be called the "stress-effect." Now, imagine tripping over that *same rock*, in exactly the same way, but this time the trip occurs while walking along the edge of a cliff, nearly throwing you over. In both scenarios, the act of tripping (the stressor) was identical. However the effect on your bodymind (the stress-effect) was dramatically different. The first trip was inconvenient; the second, terrifying!

Beginning in the 1980s, many articles were published in the world's medical literature about the interactions between various stressors and their effects on human physiology. The first article to catch my attention described British research on study participants who reported a severe allergy to corn.[19] While sitting inside a Faraday Cage, they demonstrated no allergic response to corn. Upon exiting the cage, they once again demonstrated an allergic response. It turned out that by temporarily removing the electromagnetic stressors, the participants were relieved of enough *total stress burden* that they, in effect, moved away from the cliff. (Note: No one should *ever* attempt to test serious food allergens without close medical supervision.)

Again, it is the *total load* of accumulated stressors that pushes one beyond their reserves to the point where dis-ease is manifested. In other words, each individual can accommodate stress up to a certain point. Once that individual threshold is crossed, symptoms of dis-ease appear because the body no longer has sufficient reserves to keep illness at bay.

Obviously, the closer you are to the edge of the cliff, the less you can afford to trip. Likewise, the closer you are to the limits of the functional capacity of any organ system in your body (immune, vascular, gastrointestinal, skeletal or nervous system), the less you can afford to make careless lifestyle choices. In our analogy, therefore, the onset of dis-ease can be likened to falling over the edge of the cliff. This book is designed to teach you how to *back away from the cliff*.

The most efficient and effective approach in terms of money, time and effort for moving away from the cliff is two-fold: reduce your exposure to environmental stressors wherever possible, and simultaneously, implement the 3LS into your lifestyle to increase your body's available reserves for dealing with life's unavoidable stressors. By increasing the distance between yourself and the edge of the cliff, you decrease the stress-effect of each stressor, thereby significantly lowering your total bodymind burden. In so doing, you will have a much better chance of preventing illness when you encounter life's psychosocial stressors.

Human Evolution and Adaptation

The human body tends to evolve rather quickly—both individually and collectively—to survive in this rapidly changing environment. It's amazing how rapidly modern civilizations have adapted to environmental stressors that were non-existent just two hundred years ago—as illustrated by the power lines and radio waves examples in this chapter. Likewise, the Europeans who traveled to the United States in the 1500s were more resistant to smallpox and measles than the Native Americans who had never before been exposed.

Here's another example. Less than two decades ago, the American Red Cross shipped a large supply of milk to Bangladesh as a relief effort after a devastating flood. Soon after the milk's consumption, world medical literature began reporting a startling increase in the development of secondary sexual characteristics (menstruation, breast development, pubic hair, penile and testicular growth, etc.) in Bangladesh children between the ages of five and ten. Neither these children nor their parents grew up drinking cow's milk, so as a population group, they couldn't tolerate its hormonal residuals. On the other hand, most Americans have been exposed to cow's milk for decades. Having had time to accommodate to this *particular* stressor, only a small percentage of American children have shown some of these effects (although not as dramatically nor as early in life).

The faster our environment changes, the faster humankind must find ways to adapt. Unfortunately, evolution comes too slowly for the most vulnerable members of our society. With the continuing increase in the number of significant background environmental stressors, can we really afford to wait another fifty years to integrate the principles of this book into a holistic medical approach in this country?

Now that you have the basics on the relationship between stress (both environmental and psychosocial) and chronic dis-ease, it's time to get a bit more technical. At the risk of overwhelming or intimidating some of my readers, the next chapter will delve more deeply into the mechanisms behind this process. I strongly discourage you from skipping over the material. You *can* understand this information, and the reward will be well worth the effort!

CHAPTER 6

Stored Stress-Effect and the Hypothalamus

I would feel more optimistic about a bright future for man if he spent less time proving that he can outwit Nature and more time tasting her sweetness and respecting her seniority.

~ E.B. White
(U.S. author and humorist, 1899–1985)

The Fight-or-Flight Response

Like all animals, human beings come equipped with a life-saving, automatic internal response to danger, termed the fight-or-flight (FOF) response. During the FOF response, heart and respiratory rates increase, blood flow diverts from the digestive tract to the limbs, alertness increases and pupils dilate. The FOF response served our ancestors well, giving them the strength and endurance to survive by fighting an attacker or fleeing sudden danger.

Unlike the *actual*, physical threats often faced by primitive humans, most of the encounters eliciting the FOF response in our bodies today are *perceived* threats. And since, for example, we no longer face the sabre-toothed tiger, we rarely *act* on this instinctive response in the same ways our ancestors did. It's just not socially acceptable to go around beating up our bosses, neighbors or spouses just because we feel angry with or threatened by them. Nor would it be appropriate to run out of the room during an important job interview, or flee the classroom in a panic when it's time to give a presentation.

As explained in the previous chapter, the word "stress" encompasses the psychological and social challenges of day-to-day life *as well as* the various environmental stressors that are often overlooked. When we experience the adrenaline rush of a near-miss auto accident or heated argument, the physiological effects of the FOF response in the body are obvious. Less obvious are the physiological effects that are being automatically induced by the thousands of environmental stressors we encounter every day. Why is this significant?

Consider this: Your body undergoes a physiological FOF stress response each time you encounter television and computer screens, mobile phones, microwave ovens, power lines, radio waves, pesticides, household cleaners, processed foods, artificial sweeteners and so forth. That means this primitive life-saving response is now being activated almost continuously in various degrees—a very unfortunate and counterproductive consequence of living in our high-tech world.*

Regardless of whether we physically *act* on our instincts (fight or flee) when encountering both real and perceived threats, our bodies still *automatically respond* to some degree. This is as true now as it was in ancient times. Whenever the FOF response is induced, it creates a chemical "readiness" in the system—meaning the body is physiologically *ready* to fight or flee. When not released by the physical act of fighting or fleeing, the stress-effect of this undischarged readiness accumulates and stores itself in the hypothalamus, the master endocrine gland.[2]

Hypothalamus: Home to Stress-Effect Storage

All outside stimuli are collected and interpreted by the cerebral cortex (the portion of the brain responsible for thought, reasoning, memory and voluntary movement), which in turn, is directly connected to the hypothalamus. The hypothalamus is the part of the brain that connects the activity of the cerebral cortex and the input from our environment to the functions of our bodies. Every single FOF response—no matter its cause—is mediated through the hypothalamus. In other words, what is

---

* On a positive note, that same FOF response mechanism can purposely be used for our benefit through visualization. Many athletes have discovered they can improve their game simply by visualizing themselves performing and achieving their goals.[1] In addition, the entire premise of hypnotherapy is based on this conscious and subconscious mind-body relationship, which tends to run on default until or unless we either reprogram the subconscious mind or learn to redirect it consciously.

going on in our bodies is very much a response to what is going on in our brains. Not only is the brain itself the master of the body, but the mind and body are *one* (the "bodymind").

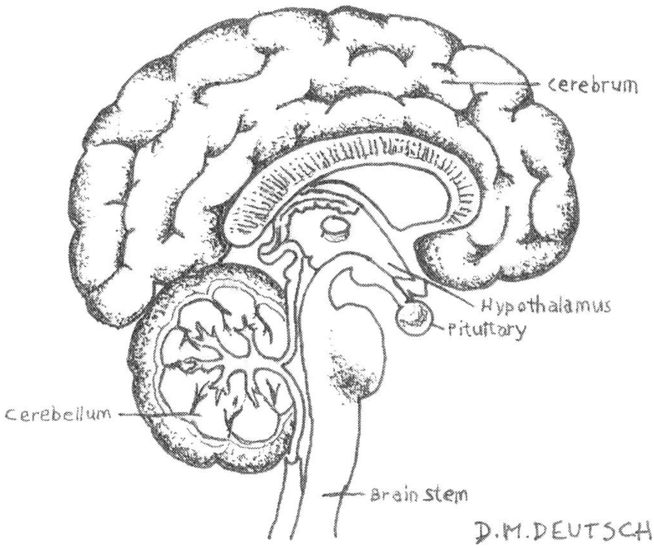

The Hypothalamus

Anything that affects a person physically, mentally, emotionally or spiritually influences every other single aspect of that person's function. The hypothalamus regulates both endocrine function and autonomic nervous system function (things like body temperature, appetite, sleep and blood pressure) either directly via the limbic system (involved with emotion and behavior); or indirectly via the hormonal effects mediated through the pituitary gland. Understanding this, you can begin to see how its hyperstimulation due to stress-effect storage is the mechanism by which "stress" causes dis-ease.

Aside from the degree, to the hypothalamus there is no difference between the stress-effect of an environmental stressor and that of a psychosocial stressor, let alone any difference between a real threat and a perceived threat. *Every* stressor evokes the FOF response in the body to a greater or lesser degree, and *every* stressor that cannot be released by physically running or fighting stores the *readiness* to do so in the hypothalamus.

> ***Adapt or perish, now as ever,***
> ***is nature's inexorable imperative.***
>
> ~ H.G. Wells (1866–1946)

If we could at least *act* on the primitive impulse of FOF every time it was being induced, there would be no detrimental effect to health. The stress-effect would be immediately discharged, preventing its accumulation in the hypothalamus. Despite the fact that most of us rarely, if ever, physically discharge the readiness does not prevent its accumulation. The burden of this undischarged stress-effect eventually produces profound changes in *all* the messages passing through the bodymind. This is the most important piece of the chronic conditions puzzle and the root of what our country's disease-care system has been missing with its one-sided, treatment-based, symptom-suppressing approach.

The "Good Old Days"

Before the Industrial Revolution beginning in the late 1700s, a good night's sleep was typically all that was needed to effectively discharge one day's worth of accumulated stress-effect in the hypothalamus. In effect, humankind woke up each morning with about as much stored stress-effect as was present the morning before. Due to the increasing environmental burdens of the last two centuries (further accelerated by the industrial, electromagnetic and chemical "revolutions"), we are now being exposed to over a thousand times more stressors per day as compared to the "good old days."

Fortunately, the human body wasn't designed for living in a completely stress-free environment, so not all sources of stress need be eliminated to enjoy perfect health. On the contrary, a moderate level of stress is actually good for you.

Primitive Human

Sabre-Toothed Tiger → FOF Response → Run/Fight → Stress-Effect Immediately Discharged

and

Good Night's Sleep → 1 Day's Worth of Stress-Effect Accumulation Is Discharged

Modern Human

Electromagnetic Stressor → FOF Response → Do Nothing → Stress-Effect Stored in Hypothalamus

and

Good Night's Sleep → Only *Some* of the Day's Worth of Stress-Effect Accumulation Is Discharged

Using the term "arousal" to mean responsiveness to stimuli, the Yerkes-Dodson Law demonstrates that "optimal task performance occurs at an intermediate level of arousal, with relatively poorer performance at both lower and higher arousal levels, creating an inverted U relationship between arousal and performance."[3] (See page 68.)

The Yerkes-Dodson Law demonstrates that the human body thrives best when arousal levels are moderate. It is capable of meeting the demands of an increased stressor load, but only to a certain point. If confronted with too many stressors continuously over time without sufficiently discharging them on a daily basis, the total accumulated load reaches a point where we lose the ability to perform efficiently (often when it is needed the most). How much stress is considered too much for any particular individual depends on a combination of that person's genetically-determined horsepower and lifestyle choices.

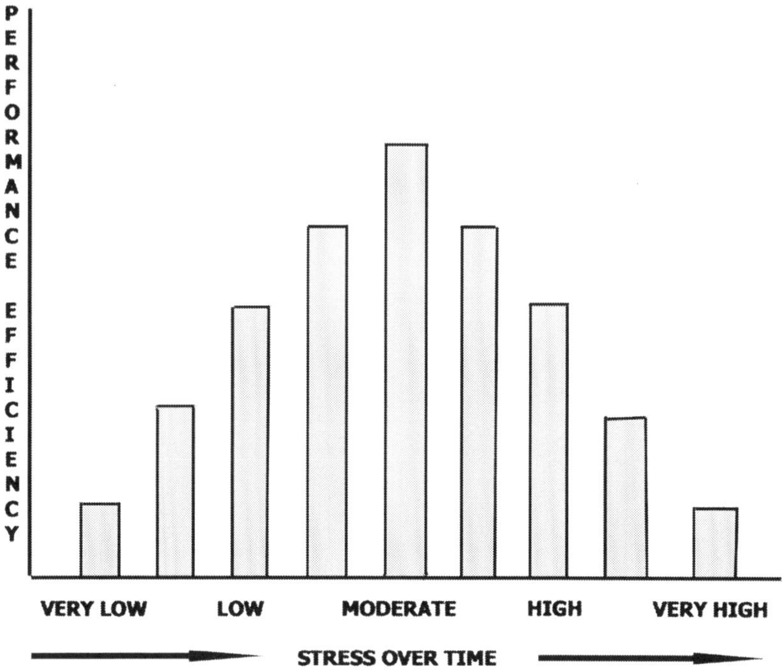

Yerkes-Dodson Law

Dr. Hans Selye (first mentioned in Chapter 5) reported rediscovering the validity of the Yerkes-Dodson Law in his classical writings about stress during the 1950s.[4] It took over fifty years for Selye's discoveries to get from his laboratory to the public. As far as I know, his teachings still haven't reached the classrooms of U.S. medical schools.

The question becomes: Since a good night's sleep is no longer sufficient to discharge one day's worth of accumulated stress-effect in the hypothalamus, how *does* it get released? Apparently, it does not. Stress-effect continues to accumulate on a daily basis until or unless we take specific actions toward discharging it.* Two of the most common manifestations

* To learn how to discharge accumulated stress-effect storage, see Chapter 24: *Skilled Relaxation.*

of hypothalamic stress-effect storage overload are decreased immunity (previously discussed) and a condition called "bracing."

Bracing: Chronic Readiness

"Bracing" is a term I use to describe chronic total-body muscle tension. Bracing is not so much something you are *doing,* but rather, something that is *happening* inside your muscles. Bracing is basically an unconscious process—the result of being in continuous FOF mode over an extended period of time.

People affected by bracing are living in bodies that are consistently ready to run and/or fight. This physiological readiness creates an abnormal level of electrical activity in each individual muscle cell twenty-four hours a day. Muscle tension accumulates, slowly and gradually, individual muscle cell by individual muscle cell. Given that bracing affects every muscle cell in the body at the same time, it can be very difficult to identify because there's no way to compare it with the rest of the body experience. Until or unless bracing leads to either chronic pain, restless legs syndrome (RLS) or any number of other tension-related symptoms, the condition tends to go virtually unnoticed.[5]

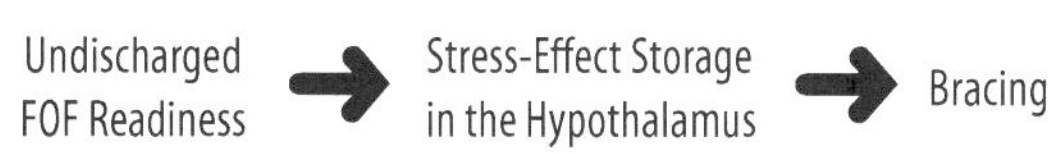

People affected by bracing often insist that they are quite "relaxed." I, too, thought I was one of the most relaxed people I knew when I first started my medical practice over forty-five years ago. I look back now and realize I was tight as a board. I had no idea that my long list of serious chronic conditions were all related to accumulated stress-effect storage and bracing. After being treated (unsuccessfully) with various pharmaceuticals for nearly ten years, I finally realized there were no magic pills for my maladies. In order to become well, I had to learn and diligently follow certain lifestyle changes, as described in Section IV of this book.

Costochondritis is a prime example of a condition most often created and made persistent by bracing. Costochondritis creates inflammation, pain and tenderness in the chest wall in the areas where the ribs attach to the intercostal muscles (the muscles between the ribs that allow your chest to expand when you breathe). So far, the only known cause of persistent tension of the intercostal muscles is bracing due to chronic stress-effect storage in the hypothalamus.*

The muscle tension inherent with bracing is constant and chronic. Being a survival mechanism, FOF limits the blood supply to areas of the body not required for fighting and fleeing. Over time, those areas of the body can no longer function optimally. For example, people affected by bracing often have cold hands and feet. After all, when the cave man was confronted with the saber-toothed tiger, the last thing he needed was for his skin to have a lot of circulation, because even minor cuts might lose a lot of blood and reduce his chances of survival.

As the next chapter will demonstrate, the bracing process also commonly diverts the blood supply from the gastrointestinal tract and directs it to the limbs, the areas most needed for fighting or fleeing. Inadequate blood supply in the gastrointestinal tract, in turn, leads to a condition known as leaky gut syndrome (LGS), a common precursor or underlying root cause of many chronic conditions.

---

* The chest pain from costochondritis can often be sharp, sometimes fooling people into thinking they are having a heart attack. Pain is worse when taking a deep breath, coughing, and with heavy exertion such as jogging or lifting.

CHAPTER 7

Leaky Gut Syndrome

Education is a progressive discovery of our own ignorance.

~ Will Durant
(American writer, historian and philosopher, 1885–1981)

LGS: If You Haven't Heard of It, You *Will*

The gastrointestinal tract (a.k.a. the G.I. tract, intestinal tract or "gut") is in fact one continuous tube that begins at the mouth and ends at the anus. Substances from the outside world (food, drink and particles you breathe in and swallow) travel through this tube in the following order: mouth, esophagus, stomach, duodenum, small intestine, large intestine (colon), rectum and anus. Notice how the inside of your mouth is, technically, outside your body. Likewise, the inside of your entire intestinal tract is also, technically, outside your body.

The previous chapter described how the accumulation of hypothalamic stress-effect storage commonly leads to a condition called "bracing." Bracing, in turn, leads to a reduced supply of blood to the intestinal tract—the organ system *least needed* in the act of fighting or fleeing. When the gut lining becomes chronically starved for blood, it will begin to function imperfectly. Eventually, it will become leaky. Of course, a gut that leaks can no longer perfectly protect your *inner* body from foreign substances originating in the *outer* world.

I estimate that more than 75% of the U.S. population has significant leakiness of the gut—a condition known as "leaky gut syndrome" (LGS). Unfortunately, since LGS is neither recognized nor acknowledged by the conventional medical paradigm, most of the affected individuals have never even heard of it. On the other hand, chiropractors, naturopaths and other holistic practitioners are *highly* aware of LGS as a major precursor to a wide variety of chronic health conditions.*

Bracing → Reduced Blood Supply to Gut → LGS → Chronic Health Conditions

To get a visual of LGS, imagine putting some fine grains of sand into a balloon, then adding some water and tying it closed. Now imagine dipping that balloon into a sink full of water. None of the sand can get into the sink *unless* the balloon has holes large enough for the grains to pass through. Likewise, in order for various ingested substances to get into your bloodstream, there would need to be holes in the protective lining of your gut large enough for *them* to pass through.

Actually, the lining of your intestinal tract does more than simply act as a shield. It also takes the substances you ingest (proteins—the "stuff of life"), breaks them down, then converts them into tiny particles that can be safely absorbed into the bloodstream (amino acids—the building blocks of protein). This includes not only food and drink, but ingested allergens and toxins as well. In order for your body to perform this process without the immune system going crazy, the intestinal lining must do its job *very* well.

When LGS is present, the gut lining's normal functions are compromised. Instead of breaking the ingested proteins all the way down into amino acids, fragments or small chains of imperfectly digested proteins, called peptides, remain hooked together. Since peptides are larger than amino acids, the only way they can enter the bloodstream is by slipping through the walls of a gut lining with large enough holes—a gut that is leaky.

Proteins → Peptides → Amino Acids

---

* If you suspect you have LGS but want proof beyond statistics and symptoms, some of the more advanced clinical laboratories offer tests to measure the permeability of the intestinal lining. One of the most common is the lactulose/mannitol test. Measured amounts of these two non-metabolized sugar molecules are given orally, followed by a six-hour urine test. The ratio of lactulose to mannitol recovered in the urine determines the relative leakiness of the gut.[1]

Peptides and the Immune System

Once peptides manage to leak through the gut walls, the immune system gets involved. In fact, many chronic conditions of conventionally "unknown" cause are due to immunological reactions to these peptides. This includes seemingly unrelated conditions such as food allergies, environmental sensitivities, arthritis, eczema, psoriasis, autoimmune disease, cancer, brain chemistry disorders, glandular problems, hormonal imbalances and even certain kinds of obesity.[2]

Basically, your immune system sees the world in black and white. When it sees something that it recognizes as *you*, all is well. When it sees something that it recognizes as *not you*, its job is to attack. Amino acids are recognized as you, peptides are not.

To further complicate the original problem, some of the peptides leaking into the bloodstream are nearly *identical* to some of the natural peptides present in the proteins of your own healthy tissues. When your immune system cannot tell the difference between the escaped peptides (what is *not* you) and the general population of your own peptides (what *is* you), the immune police (antibodies) shoot all the peptides that look the same first, and ask questions later. Of course, by then it's too late and the damage has already taken place.[3]

Leaked Peptides ➔ Immune Response ➔ Attack Everything ➔ Damage

As you might expect, the immunological reaction that occurs at the site of the leakage can also cause direct intestinal irritation. The various symptoms of this irritation are frequently diagnosed by conventional medicine as separate conditions—such as colitis, irritable bowel syndrome, Crohn's disease, ulcerative colitis, malabsorption and celiac disease (sprue)—when in fact they are all related to the same process. LGS also sets the stage for dysbiosis, an imbalance of the normal flora and a degradation of the healthy intestinal ecology.

To summarize, *localized* symptoms are often caused by the immunological reaction occurring at the site of the leakage, whereas *systemic* symptoms are caused by the immune system response to leaking peptides.

All such symptoms are presently being treated as separate diagnoses by conventional medicine when in fact they are all related to the same process—LGS.

As if holes in the gut lining and the resulting leaking peptides, immune system attacks, intestinal irritation and dysbiosis weren't enough, our bodies are also struggling to cope with a variety of relatively new man-made chemical toxins (pesticides, preservatives, toxic halides such as fluoride, bromide and chlorine, artificial additives such as flavorings, colorings and sweeteners and so forth). Since most of these toxins cannot be digested, the main way they get into the system is by passive absorption.

Toxins are handled differently by a leaky gut, making their effects more dangerous. For example, the abnormal bacterial population caused by a leaky gut tends to convert heterocyclic amines (found in processed foods) into toxic carcinogens.[4] In a vicious cycle, this combination of dysbiosis and degradation *further* aggravates LGS by increasing damage to the gut lining, thereby allowing even *more* toxic products, including carcinogens, to be absorbed into the bloodstream.[5]

Once toxins have leaked through the gut lining into the bloodstream, the next (and last) line of defense is your liver. The liver is one of the most important organs in the body. It serves many functions, including detoxifying anything harmful that escapes the gut lining and the gut-associated lymphoid tissue (the GALT, which makes up about 70% of the entire lymphoid system of the body).[6] Whether or not the liver has sufficient reserves to cope with the extra burden of toxins due to LGS is another matter.

The immune system's attack response from peptides leaking through an incompetent lining is how most environmental and food-related reactions begin. However, it is important to note that overwhelming stress-effect storage, in and of itself, can also cause immune system dysfunction (of which allergies and hypersensitivities are examples of) directly—*without* LGS. This is due to the fact that in prolonged fight-or-flight, all systems the body considers non-essential for fighting or fleeing (including the immune system) become neglected because the body is in continuous "survival" mode.

As Chapter 9 demonstrates, standard allergy testing cannot detect the processes through which the immune system responds to leaking peptides, and therefore does not officially recognize these types of "reactions." This lack of detection results in frustrated patients with a variety of confusing symptoms who are sometimes made to feel it's all in their heads. Often they are told their problem is simply "stress"—which if properly defined and understood, is an accurate assessment!

The Role of Stress in LGS

Stress, as defined in the last two chapters, plays a very big role in the long-term causation, as well as the short-term flare-ups, of all chronic disorders of the intestinal tract. After all, chronic stress (being in FOF mode) reduces blood supply to the gut, creating dysfunction.

The graph on the following page illustrates how increasing exercise intensity affects various systems of the body. Adapted from the medical physiology laboratory of the University of Kentucky School of Medicine, this graph represents the relative allocations of blood supply to various body systems at rest and with varying degrees of exercise. Since both fight and flight could be considered forms of exercise, we can use this information to infer the types of temporary changes that take place in the body when we encounter a stressor.

As you can see, no matter how intense the exercise (or stress level), blood supply to the brain remains constant. Blood supply increases most dramatically in the muscles and heart—at the expense of the gut, which suffers a dramatic decrease. When we interpret the graph in terms of chronic stress levels that result from being in continuous FOF mode, we can conclude that the farther to the right your baseline, the less blood circulation there is available to the intestinal tract twenty-four hours a day.

Every body system is vulnerable to dysfunction caused by chronic stress. The bodymind may cry out in small ways at first, then when ignored, begin to shout louder—creating more serious dysfunction. Dysautonomia (significant disturbance of the autonomic nervous system, or ANS) is a striking example. The ANS regulates our essential functions (heart rate, blood pressure, breathing, etc.) whether we are awake or asleep, conscious or unconscious. With dysautonomia, "the human body fails to properly regulate blood pressure, heart rate, temperature, vascular constriction/dilation and blood supply to the brain.

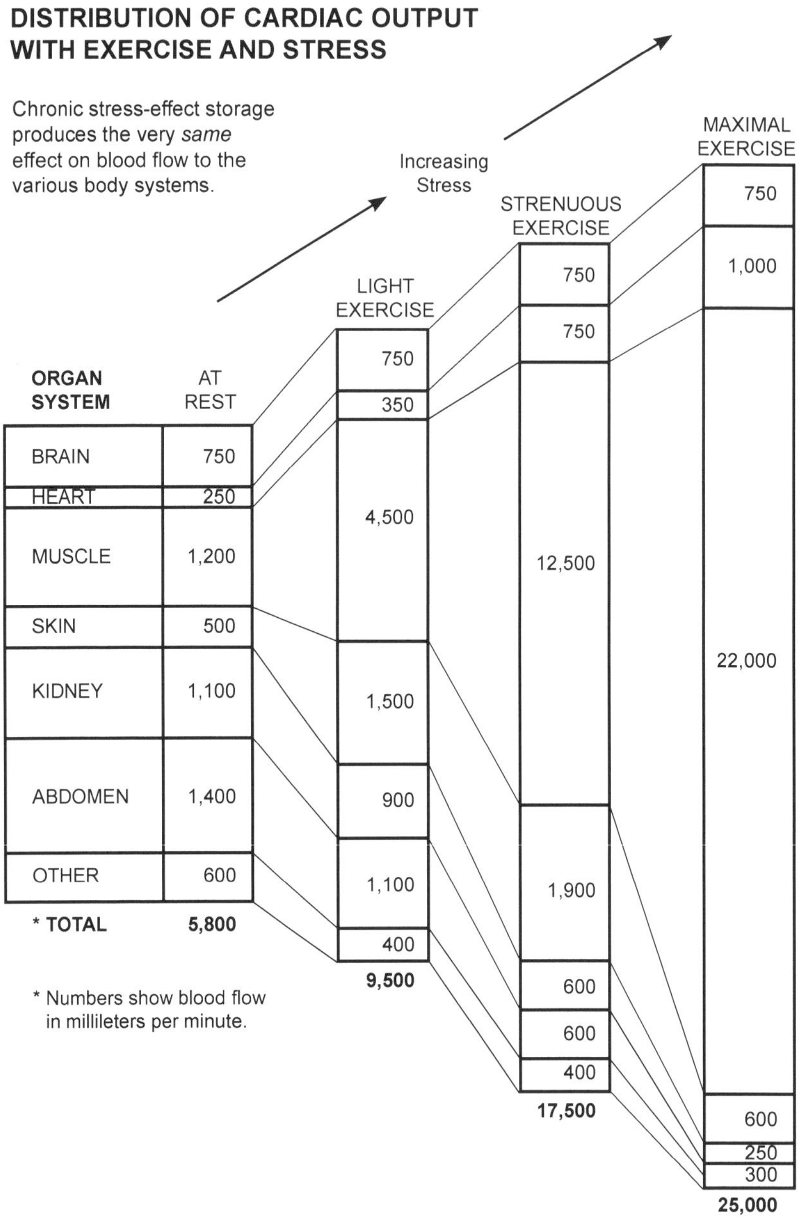

How "Stress" Affects Blood Flow

The results of dysautonomia are unpredictable fainting, extremely low blood pressure, light-headedness, dizziness, problems concentrating (brain fog), headaches, fatigue, heart palpitations, exercise intolerance, insomnia, hot flashes, chills, weakness, seizures, pain and disability."[7]

The good news is, by applying what is currently known about the physiological effects of chronic stress-effect storage, resolving most chronic health conditions can now be routine. Since it is accurate to deduce that anyone who suffers from chronic conditions has significant LGS, what then might be a logical approach for reversing these conditions at their root cause? Certainly not "treatment" via symptom-suppressive therapies!

Reversing LGS in 14 Hours (Plus 6 Months)

The lining of the entire intestinal tract replaces itself, on average, every fourteen hours. This means that in less than one day, every cell that makes up the gut lining is digested or sloughed off and a new one grown in its place. You might think, then, that healing the digestive tract can be accomplished in less than a day, but unfortunately it isn't quite that simple.

Due to its extremely fast turnover, the gut uses more blood when it is at rest than any other organ system when *it* is at rest. When stress-effect accumulates in the hypothalamus, causing blood to be diverted to the limbs, the gut is one of the first systems to be compromised. Once you succeed in normalizing the blood supply to the intestinal tract, the lining will return to normal within just fourteen hours. Yet normalizing that blood supply can take time and effort.

Since most people have accumulated a *lifetime* of stress-effect storage, it takes the average person several months of twice-a-day Skilled Relaxation (SR) to reach the point where normal blood supply to the gut even *begins* to return. A small percentage of lucky individuals can accomplish this in only three months, and most within six. However, time frames are so individual that my general recommendation is to commit to practicing SR twice daily for a year. Once LGS is healed, most people can then decrease their SR sessions to once a day for maintenance.

One indicator of progress is evidence of improved circulation to the extremities. Biofeedback research has demonstrated that as long as a person's hands are warm, there is adequate circulation to the intestinal tract.[8] Although cold hands are one of the more common indicators of

LGS, warm hands do not *necessarily* mean you are free of LGS. However, you can learn how to control hand temperature and other physiological responses through biofeedback training, which is one of many effective forms of SR.

While you are busy reversing the causes of your LGS, you can improve the function of the gut somewhat by shortening the transit time—the amount of time it takes a substance to go from the mouth, through the gut and out the anus—by including adequate fiber and water in your diet. If longstanding constipation is an issue, you may need to follow the fiber and mineral oil protocol found in Chapter 21.

In addition, there are several supplements I believe to be essential for anyone working toward reversing LGS.* First, ask your chiropractor or other alternative health care practitioner to recommend a quality digestive enzymes product (what a healthy gut would be making for itself), tailored to your individual age and circumstances. Second, LGS often creates a deficiency of the amino acid L-glutamine, so supplement this according to the directions on the label. Next, take essential fatty acids (EFAs) as described in Chapter 29.

Last but not least, probiotics are essential for helping restore a normal colonic bacterial population. Once these "friendly flora" have gotten out of balance (dysbiosis), healing the gut becomes *much* more challenging. In fact, dysbiosis makes the gut vulnerable to harmful opportunistic organisms like Candida albicans, the topic of our next chapter.

---

* Note: Wherever supplement recommendations are given throughout this book, the doses are based upon an average 150-lb. person. Individual requirements may vary.

CHAPTER 8

Candida-Related Syndrome

Never utter these words: 'I do not know this, therefore it is false.' One must study to know: Know to understand: Understand to judge.

~ Apothegm of Narada
(Ancient Hindu philosopher)

Intestinal Ecology and Dysbiosis

The previous chapter described a condition called leaky gut syndrome (LGS), detailing the mechanisms by which it is both caused and reversed. As described, an estimated 75% of the population has LGS to some extent, an unrecognized precursor to many chronic health conditions.

In the intestinal tract, there are over five hundred varieties of normal bacteria ("friendly flora") working together to keep you healthy. The job of the *normal* flora is to create conditions that are unfavorable to *abnormal* or parasitic organisms. However, once the intestinal lining becomes compromised through LGS, the ecology of the intestinal tract can easily get out of balance—a condition called dysbiosis. Dysbiosis, in and of itself, can cause a number of inflammatory responses involving the bowel, skin and connective tissues. Everyone who has ongoing LGS will eventually get some degree of dysbiosis, which in turn, can eventually lead to parasitic infestation (parasitosis).

LGS ➔ Dysbiosis ➔ Parasitosis

This chapter is about the one species of yeast most likely to cause parasitosis in humans—*Candida albicans*. The *only* thing standing between every single one of us and a parasitic infestation of Candida is a healthy intestinal ecology. As we shall see, Candida is not only a facilitator of LGS, its waste products also have a direct toxicological effect on the entire bodymind system.[1]

Candida Albicans: Yeast and Fungal Forms

There exists over a thousand species of yeast, which are simply single-celled, sugar-fermenting fungi. Common examples are baker's yeast (for making bread) and brewer's yeast (for fermenting alcohol). No earth dweller can possibly avoid the relatively harmless yeast form of Candida, given that it exists all around us and is present in everything we eat, drink, touch, smell and breathe. Only when Candida sprouts from the yeast (seed) form into its active fungal (plant) form does it become a parasitic issue.

Just as there are many acorns on the ground but few oak trees, so too, there are quadrillions of Candida seeds around, but few that succeed in sprouting. Seeds are nature's way of preserving an organism's life until it can find fertile ground. If an acorn lands on pavement, it is going to have a hard time growing. Likewise, if the yeast form of Candida lands in a healthy intestinal tract, it will have a hard time growing. A healthy bacterial gut ecology creates a very unfriendly place for the Candida seed, therefore it simply passes through and exits the body without sprouting.

Humans have lived side-by-side with this organism without incident up until the past two hundred years or so. Beginning with the Industrial Revolution, the number of environmental stressors we have had to cope with has increased dramatically. Pushed beyond the limits of our evolutionary capacity, many individuals have accumulated significant hypothalamic stress-effect storage, pushing them across that line of their immune system reserves, and rendering them unable to keep the Candida parasite at bay.

Stored Stress-Effect → Bracing → LGS → Dysbiosis → Candida Infestation

Even without pre-existing LGS, sometimes normal flora get temporarily thrown out of balance in an otherwise healthy intestinal tract; for example when a course of antibiotics is taken. Antibiotics not only kill off the disease-causing bacteria they are designed to target, but also the friendly bacterial population that protects us against additional disease-causing organisms and/or parasitic invasions. Whenever antibiotics are taken, what will happen next depends on several factors. Balance can sometimes be restored fairly easily by taking a good probiotic supplement. However, once parasitic organisms like Candida have become firmly established, probiotics alone will no longer be sufficient to reverse the problem.

Antibiotic Treatment → Dysbiosis → Candida Infestation

All fungi thrive by establishing themselves on dead or dying tissue. The less healthy the intestinal lining, the more dead or dying tissue there is available to the fungi. Once Candida establishes itself and sprouts into the fungal phase, it begins excreting metabolic toxins capable of killing any adjacent tissues that are less than vigorously healthy (partially dead). Once that adjacent tissue begins to die, the fungus can live on *it* as well, and so on.

Like all living things, parasites strive to create conditions conducive to their own survival. When Candida succeeds in sprouting into the active fungal form, it forms little roots (mycelia) that grow into the gut wall. The longer the infection is present, the deeper the roots can reach, therefore the more challenging it can be to rid yourself of the parasite.

I refer to chronic fungal Candida infestation of the gastrointestinal tract as "Candida-related syndrome" (C-RS) because this terminology better illustrates that an entire group of symptoms are frequently related to this one single cause. Unfortunately, a lack of recognition of C-RS by Western medicine leaves many patients to wonder why they feel so miserable despite being told everything is "normal."

C-RS: The Missing Diagnosis

The identification of Candida as an underlying factor in many previously unexplained chronic symptoms was first described in the late 1970s by Orian Truss, MD and published in his book, *The Missing Diagnosis*, in 1985. Since then, many books such as *The Yeast Connection* by William Crook, MD and *The Yeast Syndrome* by John Trowbridge, MD have helped increase awareness of this condition in the general public.[2] I highly recommend obtaining a copy of one or more of these books in order to find out if it was written about you.

The symptoms of C-RS are many and varied, and are mainly due to toxic waste products produced by the active (fungal) phase of this organism's metabolic processes being absorbed into the systemic blood supply. Symptoms include fatigue, depression, mood swings, cravings for carbohydrates and sweets, brain fog, bloating, gas, achy joints, sensitivities to perfumes, as well as a wide array of complaints that your doctor may be attempting to "treat" as separate diagnoses. Naturally, C-RS serves to make LGS much worse.

In one sense, discovering the Candida-illness connection may come as a relief because finally, patients who've long been suffering with a long list of bizarre, seemingly unrelated symptoms can receive an explanation more acceptable than hypochondria or "it's all in your head." In my experience, more than half of patients with chronic conditions for which conventional medicine has been unable to find a cause have undiagnosed C-RS.

Unlike chiropractors and naturopaths, very few conventional practitioners acknowledge the existence of LGS *or* C-RS. Thankfully, these processes are now beginning to be taught to some first-year medical students. Recently, even seasoned allopaths have begun to acknowledge the connection between antibiotic treatment and the more obvious yeast-related conditions like vaginal yeast infections and oral thrush, and so have at least started encouraging their patients to eat yogurt containing live active probiotic cultures both during and after antibiotic treatment.

Despite a great deal of misinformation to the contrary, any overgrowth of the Candida fungal phase always remains contained within the gastrointestinal tract. C-RS is never terminal; however, I've known many patients who have felt so sick for so long they *wished* they would die. Only when there is total failure of the immune system would the Candida organism itself be able to find its way into the bloodstream. When this occurs (very rare), it is called systemic candidiasis, a life-threatening condition that should *never* be confused with C-RS.

Limitations of Laboratory Testing

If you suspect you have C-RS, keep in mind that current laboratory testing is, unfortunately, highly unreliable. However, Candida questionnaires are available in books as well as through many online resources. In my opinion, these questionnaires provide at least as accurate a diagnosis as the best laboratory test.

If you insist on trying for a more scientific confirmation of your suspected C-RS, don't waste your time or money sending specimens to your local labs. According to my professional experience, the only two laboratories capable of accurately diagnosing the presence of Candida (and other parasites) in the colon are Genova Diagnostics and Meridian Valley Lab.[3] Even the Centers for Disease Control and Prevention in Atlanta agrees that local labs are about one-tenth as accurate at finding parasites as Genova and Meridian Lab. For example, when parasites are intentionally placed in a test specimen, local labs tend to find only one-fiftieth of them, whereas Genova finds one in five—still leaving an 80% chance that an active C-RS infection will be missed.

As you can see, false negatives are common even with the best of labs. On the other hand, there's no such thing as a false *positive* result (unless your specimen somehow got mixed up with someone else's). A positive test result means that parasites *have* been found, and the diagnosis is confirmed. Bird watching is a great analogy. When bird watchers look for a particular species of bird and are unable to find it, there are two possible reasons. It is either extinct (doesn't exist) or it simply wasn't found (was missed) on that particular day by that particular bird watcher. However, if the bird *is* seen, there can be no doubt as to its presence.

Permanent Eradication

Not surprisingly, C-RS tends to be one of the more challenging conditions to overcome. A few decades ago, the approaches that were used ignored the importance of healing the underlying leaky gut. When LGS was ignored, the average length of treatment was two years with a 90% relapse rate. We now realize that as long as LGS is present and the intestinal tract remains starved for blood, no treatment for pathogenic organisms will ever succeed in giving permanent results. Since C-RS makes LGS much worse, together they produce a vicious cycle that can only be stopped with a comprehensive approach.

If you think you have C-RS and have not already done so, go back and study the previous chapter until you fully understand LGS—what it is, how it is caused and how it can be reversed. *Only when actions are taken to heal LGS can anti-Candida treatments have a good chance of permanent success.* Once you have normalized blood supply to the gut, and taken steps to reverse dysbiosis, *then* efforts toward "treatment" for C-RS can be successful. After all, if your goal is to permanently eradicate Candida, doesn't it make sense to first create an environment unfriendly to its survival? Indeed, that is the *only* approach that can succeed in the long run.

To raise new questions, new possibilities,
to regard old questions from a new angle,
requires creative imagination
and marks new advances in science.

~ Albert Einstein (1879–1955)

Of the three legs of the 3LS of Wellness, Skilled Relaxation (SR) is by far the most important for reversing LGS. However, to be successful in eradicating Candida, incorporating Whole Foods into your diet is also extremely important. Sugars and refined carbohydrates are Candida's main food source, and must be completely eliminated during the treatment period. Since the benefits of each leg of the 3LS are multiplicative, by following all three of these lifestyle practices simultaneously, C-RS can be permanently eradicated in 3–6 months for the vast majority of patients.

Many herbal and supplemental anti-fungal formulas have been designed for combating Candida. Any of these formulas *may* be helpful as long as they are used in conjunction with the 3LS. Unfortunately, there seems to be a high incidence of people becoming either hypersensitive or resistant to such treatments over time. Therefore, my treatment of choice is pure Nystatin powder (only available by prescription). Nystatin is safe and is not absorbed from the intestinal tract. Hypersensitivities and resistance factors with Nystatin powder are so rare they can be dismissed by any reasonable consideration.

If you decide to ask your doctor for this medication, be certain your doctor does not prescribe Nystatin liquid or tablets. Both are full of sugar, Candida's source of food. Also, I have seen some inexperienced physicians make the mistake of ordering topical Nystatin powder, which is for external use and is mostly talcum powder. You want the *oral* form of pure Nystatin powder, so be sure double check with your doctor and at the pharmacy.

Much of the literature about Candida speaks of severe "die-off" (herxheimer) reactions. Symptoms such as headaches, nausea, fatigue, cravings, depression, flu-like symptoms and body aches are frequently reported during the first several days of treatment. I believe that many of the symptoms attributed to die-off are more likely a result of withdrawal symptoms that occur when switching from a refined diet to perfect Whole Foods. Be sure to study Chapters 26 and 27 so you understand how to get through the withdrawal symptoms in the shortest amount of time possible (3 4 days). Your efforts will more than pay off in the many years to come.

Section III

CHRONIC HEALTH CONDITIONS

Disease Care
Is *Not* the Solution

CHAPTER 9

Allergy and Hypersensitivity

You will observe with concern how long a useful truth may be known and exist before it is generally received and practiced on.

~ Benjamin Franklin
(Founding father of the U.S., 1706–1790)

Allergy Tests and Shots: 5% Effective!

The incidence of allergy in the United States has been increasing at the alarming rate of more than 100% over the past fifty years, and by more than 50% over the past twenty years alone, with an estimated one in five Americans suffering as of 2003. The incidence and severity of asthma, as a component of allergy, has been increasing at an even greater rate.[1] Many Americans are finding themselves in the unfortunate position of reacting to wider and wider varieties of foods, animals, plants, molds, perfumes and other substances. Are we evolving into a new race or are we simply struggling to cope with the rapid and drastic changes in our environment?

Conventional medical options for the diagnosis and treatment of allergy are still mired in the dawn of its outdated understanding from over eighty years ago. I can still remember sitting through a lecture in medical school, learning that the then-current science of allergy diagnosis and treatment was only 5% effective. In studies using the famous double-blind method, 55% of patients receiving allergy shots (twice a week for two years) reported improvement in their symptoms. That sounded promising, until we learned that 50% of patients receiving a placebo (water in a syringe) *also* reported similar improvement. The conclusion: Allergy shots were only 5% more effective than placebo!

The entire science of allergy is based on the premise that the substance from the environment to which you are allergic (when injected, eaten, inhaled or applied to the skin) stimulates the immune globulins (serum antibodies) in the blood, causing the release of histamine. And the science is accurate, insofar as it goes. It just so happens to completely *miss* the mechanism by which 95% of all reactions are occurring.

Hidden Hypersensitivities

The huge missing piece of the puzzle lies in something known as *hypersensitivities,* which cannot be detected via standard allergy testing methods. Unlike conventionally recognized allergies, which are due to *serum* sensitivities (the clear yellowish fluid present in blood), hypersensitivities are due to *tissue* sensitivities (muscle, skin, nerve and connective tissue).[2] If no IGE, IGM or IGA serum antibodies are detected, then by definition it cannot be called an "allergy." But that doesn't mean you aren't reacting!

Undetected food and environmental hypersensitivities are just one of the many "new" major health problems in this country, yet one of the least recognized by the allopathic paradigm. Conventional allergists are still using the same testing method that misses the mechanism by which 95% of all reactions are occurring. A standard allergy test cannot detect tissue hypersensitivities any more than a smoke alarm can detect a flood. They simply are not designed to do so. You might be surprised by how many of your own unexplained symptoms are related to this mechanism.

A typical scenario is as follows. You visit a conventional allergist complaining of chronic sinus problems, asthma and unexplained skin rashes. You also happen to have arthritis, constipation, brain fog and mood swings, but it doesn't occur to you to mention it because you've never associated these types of symptoms with your "allergies." The allergist performs a panel of skin testing for the usual environmental allergens (grasses, animal dander, molds, etc.) as well as the common food allergens (milk, wheat, eggs, etc.). You test positive for grasses and mold, but are told you don't have any food allergies. You begin to wonder if your food-related reactions were all in your head.

After a year of weekly allergy shots you show little, if any, improvement. You then come across this book or stumble upon an article about hidden food hypersensitivities, and decide to conduct a therapeutic trial elimination of wheat and dairy from your diet.* Within just two weeks, you are amazed to find that not only did your "allergy" symptoms clear up, you also saw dramatic improvement in your arthritis, constipation, brain fog and mood swings.[3]

> ***The outcome of any serious research can only be to make two questions grow where only one grew before.***
>
> ~ Thorstein Veblen (1857–1929)

When it comes to *food,* the main difference between an allergy and a hypersensitivity, both subjectively and objectively, is that food hypersensitivities tend to be extremely complex and can be much more difficult to distinguish. With a food *allergy,* reactions are typically black and white, cut and dry, obvious and immediate. But with a food *hypersensitivity,* any number of complex combinations is possible.[4] You might react to wheat only when you've had potatoes the day before (or even as many as three days before). You might react to dairy only when you've had wheat and rice during the same meal. The reaction symptoms may not be as obvious, either. With a hypersensitivity, you may experience headache, fatigue or an exacerbation of any number of chronic conditions from which you already suffer.

Clinical ecologists, who are certified by the American Academy of Environmental Medicine, are trained to look for both serum *and* tissue sensitivities. These experts in environmental and chemical sensitivities have been trying to get the field of allergy to acknowledge the 95% of reactions they are missing with their serum-only testing. Theron Randolph, MD was the first U.S. expert in the specialty of clinical ecology to explain the process of tissue sensitivities, which he called "clinical ecological tissue-specific sensitivities" (CETSS).[5]

The fact that most Americans have never even heard of clinical ecology is a perfect example of how the almighty dollar is calling most of the shots in our disease-care system. The field of allergy has actually sponsored bills in several states attempting to *outlaw* clinical ecology. Could it be because the only laboratory available for testing for tissue sensitivities

---

* See Chapter 26: *Whole Foods* and Chapter 27: *Elimination/Provocation Diet.*

is one's own bodymind, and the only effective treatment is lifestyle modification, neither of which can be patented and sold?

The defining mechanism of both allergy *and* hypersensitivity is an overreaction by the immune system to a perceived threat. Although the *mechanism* of allergies differs from that of hypersensitivities, when it comes to food reactions, both allergies and hypersensitivities are immune responses to the *protein* of the food. Both can, in rare instances, lead to a life-threatening reaction known as anaphylactic shock.*

Is Your Immune System Confused?

As described in detail in Chapter 7, leaky gut syndrome (LGS) plays a central role in immune system dysfunction. Once a foreign substance leaks into your bloodstream, it is considered a threat (antigen) to the body. The immune system's natural response is to make antibodies that are shaped in such a way as to perfectly fit the specific antigen, like a puzzle. When the antibody unites with the antigen, the antigen is neutralized. This immune response can be either *helpful* (such as providing immunity to a disease) or *harmful* (such as causing a reaction to a food).

Protein is the "stuff of life." Every living thing contains, within the actual living parts of its molecular makeup, proteins that are unique to its own particular species—and food is no exception. The two most common dietary proteins that create food-related reactions are casein and gluten (the proteins found in milk and wheat), neither of which were commonly eaten by our earliest ancestors.[6] Other foods that commonly cause reactions include peanuts, tree nuts, eggs, corn, fish, shellfish and soybeans.

Intestinal permeability due to LGS is significant, whether you are dealing with food or any other type of environmental reaction. For example, nearly 100% of inhaled environmental substances end up in the intestinal tract, by being trapped in the mucus and carried (via cleansing cilia) into the laryngeal/esophageal junction where they are swallowed. A normal, healthy gut lining can take care of these substances; a leaky gut generally cannot.

When cellular antibodies—originally designed to attack these "faux invaders"—start also attacking any matching peptides in your *own* body

* Anyone who is at risk for this type of neurogenic shock reaction should have epinephrine immediately available for self-administration by injection at all times.

tissues, the unfortunate result is a confused immune system that cannot tell the difference between what is *you*, and what is *not you*. Since every part of the bodymind has protein as part of its makeup, every single body system can be affected (and become symptomatic) via this process.

Lightening the Total Load

The following graph gives an example of a male with a family history of allergies who happens to be allergic to wheat. He doesn't view his allergy as severe, so he indulges in wheat-containing foods like bread and pasta on occasion and just deals with the consequences. On the graph, the "threshold" is analogous to the cliff described in Chapter 5. The thicker the arrow, the more intense the reaction to any additional stressor.

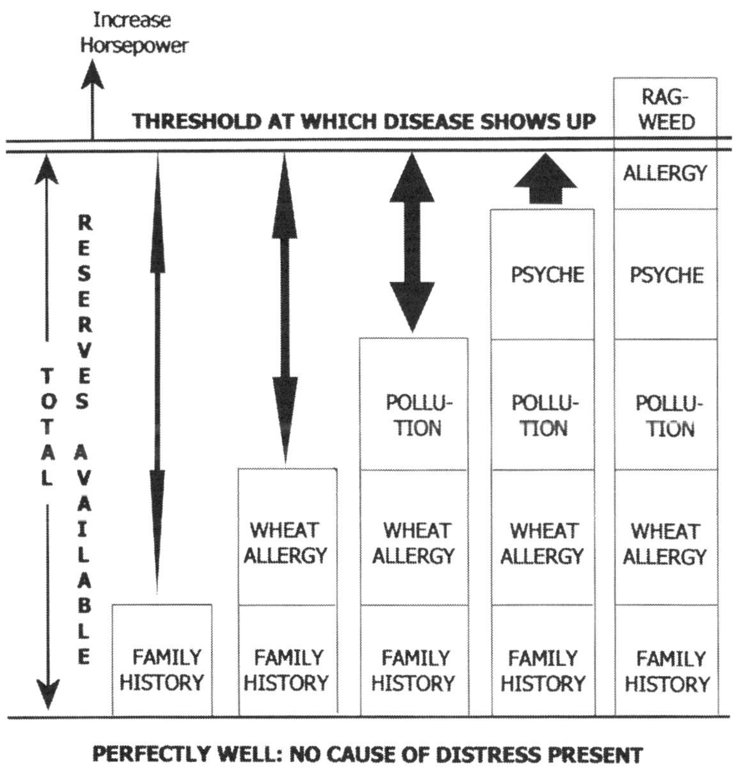

Allergy Example of Stress Response

This person's family history would indicate that he was born closer to the limits of his immune reserves than the average person. Yet he feels fine until it's "that time of year" when ragweed pollen matures and is blown into the air. Desensitizing allergy shots and antihistamine drugs help alleviate his hay fever (allergic rhinitis) symptoms during ragweed season, but do nothing about the fact that he is so close to the threshold of dis-ease (the edge of the cliff) that it only takes *one* additional stressor (ragweed season) to push him into becoming symptomatic.

If he truly wanted to eliminate his hay fever symptoms during ragweed season, he could approach it in one of two ways. He could eliminate all traces of wheat from his diet just before and during ragweed season (thus lowering his total stressor burden to the point where he would likely be asymptomatic). Or, he could take steps to increase his horsepower (raise his level of overall health and therefore his threshold) by following the 3LS Wellness protocol described in Section IV of this book. Of course, combining *both* approaches is the most effective, and prudent, thing to do.

Elimination of *any* of the stressors graphed would accomplish the same result as dietary elimination of wheat. However, it is far more difficult to eliminate things like pollution and genetic predispositions. My entire philosophy is based on finding effective holistic approaches for relief of suffering in the short term, while at the same time, implementing a Wellness lifestyle for prevention and/or reversal of disease in the long term.

Since both allergies and hypersensitivities involve immune system dysfunction, once a person with a genetic predisposition for these conditions "falls over the cliff," more serious autoimmune disorders can develop. The term "autoimmune" refers to a variety of conditions in which the immune system begins attacking the body's own tissues. Examples include multiple sclerosis (MS), eczema, psoriasis, rosacea, Graves' disease, lupus erythematosis, scleroderma, rheumatoid arthritis, and a whole host of other conditions far too numerous to list.

Short-Term Relief, Long-Term Cure

If you believe this chapter was written about you, consider seeing a clinical ecologist. Since nearly all clinical ecologists are also board-certified allergists, you'll get the best of both worlds by scheduling a consultation.

If you have already been to a conventional allergist, bring a copy of all your records to avoid the expense of repeating any tests.

In the meantime, you can get started implementing the 3LS Wellness guidelines outlined in Section IV of this book and experiment with nutritional supplementation in addition to any medications you may be taking. True allergic reactions involve the release of histamine, thus the popularity and effectiveness of antihistamine medications. Vitamin C also has an antihistamine effect and is perfectly safe, relatively inexpensive and has many positive side benefits such as boosting the immune system. I recommend taking esterified vitamin C to tolerance for one week, followed by the correct maintenance dose for your individual system. Additionally, most patients who have asthma as a complication of their allergies are deficient in magnesium, so correcting the deficiency will often greatly reduce the need for anti-asthmatic drugs.*

Of course, the most effective *short-term* approach for relieving the symptoms of allergies and hypersensitivities is to identify and eliminate the offending substances. When it comes to food hypersensitivities, use your bodymind as the laboratory. Conducting an elimination/provocation diet will help you clearly identify which dietary proteins are causing your symptoms.**

Once identified, it takes discipline and diligence to continue your complete and total avoidance of *all traces* of the offending dietary substances long enough for the immune system to "forget" how to make that particular antibody (about six months for most people). To remain mindful of your long-term goal and motivated to stick to your plan each and every day, consider posting a six-month calendar on your wall. Note any exciting improvements in your health, crossing each day off as you go.

---

* Instructions on taking vitamin C to tolerance and determining your correct maintenance dose can be found in Chapter 10: *Recurrent Colds and Flu*. Instructions for identifying and correcting magnesium deficiency can be found in Chapter 28: *Intracellular Magnesium*.

** For information on *why* dietary elimination must be "perfect," see Chapter 26: *Whole Foods*. For instructions on *how* to properly eliminate offending food proteins, see Chapter 27: *Elimination/Provocation Diet*.

CHAPTER 10

Recurrent Colds and Flu

The art of medicine consists of amusing the patient while nature cures the disease.

~ Voltaire
(French writer and philosopher, 1694–1778)

Colds and Flu Are *Not* Inevitable

For most people, occasional colds and flu ("influenza") are accepted as a fact of life. Adults in this country contract an average of three colds per year, and children an average of six. Before I became familiar with holistic medicine, I suffered my fair share of frequent colds and flu. As a family practice physician, I considered these viruses to be one of the inevitable risks of my profession, a sort of "occupational hazard."

The typical duration of the common cold is between 7–14 days. Symptoms include runny nose, sneezing, sore throat, headache, mild fatigue and sometimes a slight fever or mild cough. Flu comes on more suddenly, lasts longer and includes a more severe version of the just-listed cold symptoms along with higher fever, chills and/or sweating, cough, extreme fatigue and significant body aches.

Prevention and treatment methods given today are the very same ones I learned back in medical school. For prevention: Avoid exposure to sick individuals, cover your face when you cough or sneeze and wash your hands frequently. For treatment: Get extra rest, drink plenty of fluids and suppress any bothersome symptoms with decongestants, antihistamines and anti-inflammatory drugs. Like everyone else, I was waiting for the "cure for the common cold" to be discovered.

This chapter describes several missing critical factors, none of which I was exposed to during my conventional training. Your first goal is *prevention*—meaning, you want to avoid "catching" colds and flu in the first place. Not surprisingly, the most important underlying factor in preventing *any* illness is the strength of your immune system, and the very best way to improve your immunity is by practicing the 3LS Wellness protocol as outlined in Section IV of this book.

The next critical preventive factor is proper humidification of indoor air. One of the main reasons people come down with more colds and flu in the winter isn't due to exposure to the cold temperatures *outside* (although any stressor to the body can decrease immunity), it's due to the low relative humidity *inside*, affecting the air we breathe in our homes, schools and workplaces. The problem is, all inspired air must be 100% humidified by the time it reaches your lungs.*

Humidification: Why It Matters

In order for cold and flu viruses to enter your bloodstream, they must first penetrate the mucous lining of your respiratory tract. A normal respiratory tract makes over a quart of mucus every twenty-four hours (which explains why you swallow involuntarily every few minutes).[1] All this mucus serves two important purposes: to humidify the air you inhale, and to trap airborne invaders like viruses, bacteria and allergens. Once trapped in the mucus, tiny cilia that line the respiratory tract simply sweep these invaders into the stomach where they are easily destroyed by the powerful acid produced there.

Sound efficient? It really *is*. When everything is working as it should, the invaders don't stand a chance of penetrating the lining of your mucous membranes and causing illness. Of course, drinking plenty of

---

* Moisture from warm air always condenses on cold surfaces, just as condensation forms on the outside of a cold pitcher of lemonade in the summer. Following this same principle, condensation will form along the inside of the exterior walls of a heated and insulated building during the winter season, lowering the average indoor humidity to only about 10%. That's even drier than the average 25% humidity of the Sahara Desert!

water not only helps this process run efficiently, but is an effective preventive measure against dis-ease in and of itself.*

Extremely low humidity levels rapidly dry out and thicken your mucus. The thicker the mucus, the more slowly it will flow through your respiratory tract into your stomach. The slower it flows, the more time invading organisms will have to penetrate the lining of your mucous membranes and enter your bloodstream. Given these facts, the importance of restoring proper humidity levels inside our buildings during the winter heating season cannot be overestimated.

Research has shown an astonishing 80% reduction of viral respiratory infections in children who attend schools with heating system humidifiers.[2] To enjoy similar benefits at home, consider installing a whole-house cool mist humidifier, setting the humidistat between 40–50%. When calculating the cost of a whole-house system, several factors must be considered. Humidified air feels warmer than dry air, so you will be able to set your thermostat between 3–8 degrees lower, thereby saving money on your heating bill. Next, humidification greatly reduces air-borne allergens, helping allergy sufferers sleep much more soundly. Better sleep alone boosts immunity. As a bonus, you can expect to save significant money on doctor's fees, medications and sick days taken from work.

If installing a whole-house system isn't an option, consider running a large portable cool-mist humidifier in every bedroom, twenty-four hours a day, locating the unit near the head of the bed while you sleep. Although steam vaporizers are also effective, cool-mist humidifiers put more total moisture into the air and are the most cost-effective of the portable unit varieties. Both types serve to help moisten the mucus so nature can do its job.

Keep in mind the immune system doesn't need to come into play until *after* an invading organism has made it through the mucous lining and into the bloodstream. Once the invaders *do* succeed, whether you get sick or stay well depends on the strength of your immune system. Recent research shows that both vitamin D and C levels play a key role.

---

* The number of ounces of pure water you ideally need per day (not counting any other liquids you may be drinking) equals half your body weight in pounds. For example, a person weighing 150 pounds would drink about 75 ounces of water per day.

Vitamin D: Are You Deficient?

Adequate vitamin D levels are crucial to the health of the immune system. "In the largest and most nationally representative study of the association between vitamin D and respiratory infections ... study participants with the lowest vitamin D blood levels—less than 10 mg per milliliter of blood—were about 40% more likely to report having a recent respiratory infection than were those with vitamin D levels of 30 or higher."[3]

Vitamin D is naturally produced within the body when the skin is exposed to sunlight. People with light skin synthesize approximately 20,000 IU of vitamin D simply by exposing most of their body to sunlight for twenty minutes. People with darker skin require more time in the sun to achieve similar results. During the winter season, many people become vitamin D deficient due to a combination of staying indoors and being more heavily clothed when outdoors.

Unfortunately, the media and the sunscreen manufacturers have most of the population terrified of sun exposure, blaming it for skin cancer, premature aging and so forth.* Sunscreen not only blocks the body's natural ability to manufacture vitamin D from the sun's rays, most formulas also happen to be loaded with toxic, carcinogenic substances. In addition, sunscreen has the perverse effect of filtering out the tanning ability more than the cancer-causing rays. Since dark skin in and of itself is *protective* against sun damage, using sunscreen can actually increase the risk of the very things it claims to prevent.[4]

Given the information presented thus far, it's no surprise that the "flu season" correlates with the winter season. In addition to being the time of year people are breathing the driest indoor air, it is also the time of year when people get the least vitamin D from sun exposure. Since there is very little vitamin D in the food supply, some experts are now recommending supplementing with 4,000–5,000 IU of vitamin D3 (not D2) per day

---

* Sun damage can be prevented most effectively by taking 1000 IU of natural vitamin E (mixed tocopherols) a few hours before exposure, and twice a day for 24 hours thereafter. For added protection, take 2 grams of esterified vitamin C twice a day before *and* after exposure. For severe burns, take at least 4 grams of esterified vitamin C immediately after exposure and every 4 hours thereafter, along with 1000 IU of vitamin E immediately after exposure and twice a day thereafter. Vitamin E creams are also beneficial.

during the winter season to maintain adequate blood levels. These dosage amounts are completely safe. In fact, it is now believed you would have to take 40,000 IU per day over a long period of time before there would be any risk of toxicity.[5]

The next important nutrient is vitamin C. Vitamin C not only helps *prevent* these viral illnesses by boosting immunity, it has the added potential to actually *reverse* illness once it begins. Esterified vitamin C—a form so advanced over the regular molecule that it has been patented—has the ability to get *four times* more vitamin C into the white blood cell per gram than regular vitamin C.[6]

Vitamin C: Prevents *and* Reverses Illness

As with all infectious illness, cold and flu viruses stimulate the activity of the white blood cells—your immune system's attempt to "fight off" the invader. An elevated white blood cell count, in turn, greatly increases your body's immediate demand for vitamin C. The goal is to take enough vitamin C to put the interferon "factories" (cells that inhibit viral replication) into overdrive, in effect "supercharging" your white blood cells.

The best way to determine the correct dose of esterified vitamin C for *you* is to determine your personal "bowel tolerance"—the highest dose your body can absorb before developing loose stools. Since your body uses much more of this vitamin when fighting off infection, you will need to establish two separate tolerance levels—one for prevention when you are well (the maintenance dose) and another for reversal when you are ill (the therapeutic dose).

To determine your individual *maintenance* dose, take 1–2 grams of esterified vitamin C every thirty minutes until you suddenly develop loose stools. (For a child, give half that amount every thirty minutes.) Keep track of the total number of grams it took to reach that point, subtracting the last dose just taken. Then, take half that amount twice per day.

To determine your individual *therapeutic* dose for when you are ill, at the very first sign of symptoms, follow that same process. Keep in mind it will take many more grams to reach bowel tolerance when you are battling an illness. Once you experience the loose stools , stop dosing for 3–4 hours. Then, take one quarter of that *total* amount four times per day for the duration of the viral episode. To ensure the infection is completely gone, continue at this dose for an additional twenty-four hours after your last symptom has disappeared, then go back to taking your maintenance dose.

As soon as cold and flu season begins, take your maintenance dose daily for prevention. Then, if you feel yourself starting to "come down with something," *immediately* increase to your therapeutic dose for treatment. This will often enable the immune system to arrest the virus within 24–48 hours. Best results for complete reversal will occur if the therapeutic dose is started *as soon as the first symptoms are noticed*. The longer you wait, the more time the virus has to take hold.

To illustrate the process of establishing bowel tolerance, let's say you feel yourself coming down with a cold. You immediately begin taking 2 grams of esterified vitamin C every thirty minutes. Just after your ninth dose (having taken a total of 18 grams), you run to the bathroom with loose stools. This means you were able to tolerate 16, but not 18, grams. Your total daily therapeutic dose would then be 16 grams per day (taken as 4 grams, four times per day). Once you have completely recovered, you repeat this same process. This time, loose stools develop after only 8 grams, meaning your maintenance dose is about 6 grams per day (taken as 3 grams, twice per day).

Individual tolerance levels vary *widely*. I have seen people tolerate as much as 40 grams of esterified vitamin C per day when ill and 25 grams per day when healthy. Conversely, I have seen people tolerate as little as 10 grams per day when ill and 1 gram per day when healthy. My personal tolerance levels are 4 grams per day for prevention and 24 grams per day for treatment. There's no need to worry about "overdosing" on vitamin C. The only side effect of taking too much is loose stools (harmless and temporary so feel free to experiment).

Next, two holistic treatments worth mentioning are zinc formulas and nasal irrigation. Each work via different mechanisms to prevent and/or reverse colds and flu.

Zinc and Nasal Irrigation

Research indicates that the average severity and duration of a cold can be cut by more than half by using ionized zinc formulas containing the active ingredients zinc gluconate, zinc aceticum or zincum gluconicum. A number of randomized double-blind placebo studies support these claims.[7] Zinc formulas are available over the counter at most drug stores, both as nasal formulas and oral lozenge or spray preparations.* Use as directed on the package, starting within the first twenty-four hours of cold symptoms appearing, and continuing for another forty-eight hours after all symptoms have gone.

Nasal irrigation is a safe holistic tool that has only positive benefits both in the prevention and treatment of respiratory illnesses. Nasal irrigation involves pouring warm saline water into one nostril while allowing it to flow out the other, helping clear the sinuses of things such as bacteria, viruses, allergens, pollutants, smoke and other irritants.[8] It also moistens and thins the mucus lining the respiratory tract, aiding the tiny cilia that sweep the mucus into the stomach. Its many benefits include reversing an oncoming cold, relief of allergies and relief of sinus pain and pressure. Nasal irrigation has been popular in ayurvedic and yogic traditions for over a thousand years, but most Americans were unaware of it until very recently. In 2007, the Oprah Winfrey Show featured regular guest Dr. Oz touting the benefits of the Neti pot—a small container designed for this purpose.

Now that we have covered the most effective holistic prevention and treatment methods, let's explore some of the most common conventional approaches to these types of respiratory illnesses: decongestant medications, antibiotics and flu shots.

Decongestants, Antibiotics and Flu Shots

Oral decongestants are not recommended. They tend to be ineffective and carry risks of side effects, such as affecting blood pressure. However, *topical* decongestants containing the medication oxymetazoline hydrochloride 0.05% can be very useful. Spray in each nostril as directed, and be sure to sniff hard (never blow). These types of nasal sprays prevent pressure from building up by keeping the sinus passages open, enabling the necessary drainage to occur. This, in turn, helps prevent secondary bacterial infections, thus avoiding unnecessary antibiotic treatment.

* There have been some reports of individuals losing their sense of smell after using zinc nasal formulas. The instructions are to swab the product just inside the nostril edges. Avoid inserting the product deeper into the nose or sniffing hard after application. To avoid this risk altogether, use oral zinc formulas.

Speaking of antibiotics, I continue to be dumbfounded by the fact that much of the population still doesn't understand that antibiotics are *worthless* against any and all viral illnesses, and that includes colds and flu. It's as I've always said to my patients: "If treated with antibiotics, the common cold will clear up in about ten days; and without treatment, it will clear up in about a week and a half!" In other words, the virus will run its course, with or without (the interference of) antibiotic treatment.

Flu shots were originally intended only for the elderly and those with compromised immune systems. Now they are being touted by the pharmaceutical companies, in conjunction with the Centers for Disease Control (CDC), as something nearly *everyone* should partake of annually. The 2009–2010 "swine flu scare" and its subsequent push for more and more vaccinations had me gritting my teeth.[9] In my opinion, the same goes for the recent push of Gardasil vaccines to girls and young women for the supposed prevention of HPV cervical cancer, and more recently to boys and young men for the prevention of genital warts and the risk of spreading HPV to women. Already, several deaths and severe disabilities have been reported from these vaccines. Rarely is the public informed of the many potential risks, not only of the vaccinations themselves, but of their toxic additives such as formaldehyde and thimerosal.[10]

I personally have not gotten a flu shot since 1965, despite my severe, familial, insulin-dependant diabetes. I stopped getting them once I began suspecting the AMA had non-medical motives for pushing them. This was even before I became educated about the flu shot risks just mentioned, and before I experienced the effectiveness of the 3LS Wellness lifestyle as an alternative. Flu shots are not the only thing I recommend avoiding when it comes to this chapter's topic. Two other factors make everything worse for the respiratory tract, both of which are worth mentioning here.

The Two Major "Don'ts"

The first major "don't" is: When you have an upper respiratory tract infection or suffer from allergies (the very conditions that make you want to blow your nose), *don't blow your nose!* Swelling caused by these conditions tend to block the tiny drainage openings (called ostia) to the sinuses and Eustachian tubes. Since ostia are about the diameter of the tip of a ballpoint pen, it takes very little swelling to block them. Remember the little cilia whose job it is to sweep all the mucus from the respiratory tract into the stomach? They are continuously working to keep the fluid moving out of these tiny drainage openings.

Depending on how much swelling is present when you blow your nose, it can take up to twelve hours for the fluid to move back to where it was before you blew. By blowing your nose just twice a day, forcing fluid back into the sinuses and ears each time, you are actually perpetuating your symptoms by making normal drainage impossible and greatly increasing your chances of developing a secondary bacterial infection. *Sniffing* is much healthier than blowing.

The second major "don't" is: *Don't smoke, and don't allow yourself or your children to breathe in second-hand smoke.* If you do smoke, none of the suggestions in this chapter will work as effectively. Smoking is a powerful producer of free radicals (which accelerate the aging process, including promoting premature wrinkles and baldness). Although vitamin C is one of the best antioxidants for neutralizing these free radicals, it takes about 1,000 mg (1 gram) of vitamin C to neutralize the free radicals contained in each pack of cigarettes smoked.

Cigarettes also paralyze the little cilia I keep mentioning, with each cigarette smoked paralyzing the cilia for at least an hour. After many years of this abuse, the cilia simply begin to die. Cilia death is one of the mechanisms that lead to emphysema in smokers—and in passive smokers. Research shows that five-sixths of the amount of nicotine found in the urine of the smoker is also found in the urine of the family members (including children) who live with them.[11]

And finally, this chapter would not be complete without addressing three bothersome symptoms that often accompany colds and flu: fever, sore throat and persistent cough.

Fever: Nature's Immune Response

Many people do not realize that the temperature of the human body varies throughout the day. The average normal oral temperature is 97.6 degrees upon arising in the morning, 98.6 around 1:00 P.M. and 99.6 upon retiring in the evening. Since this is an average, it can vary as much as a degree either way for any individual.

When young children (up to age 4 or 5) become ill, it is not unusual for them to run fairly high fevers. Although frightening for the parents, most doctors don't become too concerned until the temperature reaches 106.0, unless the child is known to be susceptible to seizures (then 104.0). I don't normally recommend attempting to lower a fever that is below 102 degrees, because for every degree of elevation above normal, *up to* 102.0, immunity increases about 10%. In other words, the fever helps fight off the infection. However, immunity begins to *decrease* once body temperature exceeds 102.0 degrees.

Sponging while sitting in a tepid (room temperature) bath is an effective way to reduce body temperature and has none of the risks of medications such as aspirin, acetaminophen and ibuprofen. Avoid ice packs and cold sponging. Not only are they extremely uncomfortable and stressful to the body, they're also far less effective than tepid sponging. Sponging with rubbing alcohol should *never* be done. If tepid sponging isn't possible, fever-reducing medications are a valid option. If body temperature is going up rapidly, you may want to administer the medication at 101 degrees because it takes some time to kick in.*

Sore Throat and Persistent Cough

Sore throats commonly accompany the first several days of colds and flu. The vast majority of sore throats are viral in nature. A persistent sore throat needs to be cultured for streptococcus, a bacterial infection that *does* indicate antibiotic treatment. For pain, salt water gargles are a safe and effective way of relieving sore throat pain as well as speeding healing. The warm salt water brings added immune response to the area, much like the hot compresses described in Chapter 31 bring for skin infections. The exact proportion of salt to water is very important: one-quarter teaspoon unrefined sea/mineral salt to eight ounces hot water. Too much salt causes irritation, and not enough salt causes swelling of the delicate throat tissues. Gargle as often as desired for symptomatic relief.

---

* Due to the risk of Reye's Syndrome, never give aspirin to a feverish child. Use ibuprofen or acetaminophen instead.

Coughing can be one of the most persistent and annoying symptoms of a respiratory illness. Often a cough will persist long after all other symptoms of a cold or flu have passed. If there is no fever, the mostly likely cause of a lingering cough is the act of coughing itself. Once a virus has run its course, the mechanical irritation of repeated coughing can continue a cough for weeks on end. In other words, *coughing perpetuates more coughing*. If you are left with a persistent, dry cough, focus your attention on voluntarily suppressing it (resist the urge to cough) and refrain from vocalizing (talking, singing and especially yelling) as much as possible. Humidify the air you breathe, and run a hot shower in a closed bathroom while breathing in the intense volume of steam for about ten minutes before going to bed.

Despite the many useful suggestions in this chapter, when it comes to preventing colds and flu, *nothing is more important than improving your immune system reserves*. If you sprayed a room full of people with a heavy dose of flu viruses, only about one-third of them will actually get sick.[12] The conventional paradigm will look at the third that got sick and focus on the germ theory of disease. The holistic paradigm will ask, "What is different about the two-thirds who remained well?" That difference, of course, lies in the strength of their individual immune systems.

Whether you were born with a relatively weak or a relatively strong immune system, you can improve your immunity by following the 3LS Wellness guidelines outlined in Section IV of this book. When you do, don't be surprised when you find yourself enjoying a new reputation as someone who never gets sick, even when everyone else around you *is*. They'll say you are "lucky" (but you'll know better).

CHAPTER 11

Recurrent Ear Infections

Antibiotic therapy is not an effective treatment against otitis media and rates of recurrent infections are significantly higher in children who have been treated with antibiotics.

~ *Journal of the American Medical Association* (12/18/91)

Otitis Media

Otitis media is the technical name for middle ear infections so common in young children. Although ear infections technically belong in the category of "acute" health conditions, they can also be considered "chronic" in the sense that many children suffer one episode after the other. Part of the problem lies in the fact that the sinuses and Eustachian tubes of young children are not yet well developed and, given their anatomy, fluid can easily become trapped.

In a healthy ear, the space in the middle ear (behind the eardrum) is filled only with air, allowing for normal sound transmission. Upper respiratory tract infections such as colds and flu, as well as allergies and food hypersensitivities, can cause the lining of the nasopharynx (the passage connecting the nasal cavity to the back of the throat) and by extension, the Eustachian tubes (the channel connecting the nasopharynx to the middle ear) to swell. Once the Eustachian tubes become obstructed from the swelling, the body tries to absorb the air, thus creating a vacuum. The vacuum then draws serum (a clear yellowish fluid) out of the blood to fill this space. Serum gets trapped in the middle ear, creating a perfect culture medium for infectious germs. When germs start to grow in the serum, white blood cells are drawn to the area to fight off the infection.

This combination creates "pus," which then creates pressure and pain inside the eardrum—an ear infection.

Drainage, Pressure and Infection

Any area of the body that is normally supposed to drain, but cannot, will eventually become infected. Sometimes nature's way of resolving a middle ear infection is to allow the eardrum to rupture spontaneously from the build-up of pressure—something that sounds far worse than it actually is. With spontaneous rupture of the eardrum, the pus erupts to the *outside* of the body, perfectly safe and even therapeutic. The same type of rupture *inside* the body—such as a ruptured appendix—would be a disaster.

Myringotomy is a surgical procedure that ruptures the eardrum via surgical incision. Both spontaneous and surgical ruptures do exactly the same thing—relieve the build-up of pressure by releasing fluid and pus. Once the middle ear space can drain, albeit through the perforated drum, the terrible pain subsides, and the infection rapidly heals. Children with repeated infections often get "tubes" surgically placed in their ears—called a tympanostomy. These "tubes in the ears" serve to mechanically keep the space in the middle ear open for a period of time, allowing for drainage and fewer infections.

It's nearly impossible for a physician to tell the difference between a viral and a bacterial infection just by looking in the ear, especially in young children. I recall the days when I treated all my otitis media patients with both antibiotics and oral decongestants, neither of which I now consider safe or effective for this problem. I cringe when I think back on how my own children would have been much better off not following my medical advice, but I simply didn't know any better.

Antibiotics Versus Placebo

Repeated articles in medical literature have proven that when it comes to otitis media, antibiotics are no more effective than a placebo. The fact that patients notice relief while taking antibiotics for ear infections does *not* prove that the antibiotic did any of the healing! In fact, studies have shown that 80–90% of all otitis media infections—whether viral *or* bacterial—will resolve on their own.[1] In fact, as stated in the quote that begins this chapter, children who receive antibiotics run a higher risk of repeated infections than those who do not. If ear infections have become a chronic problem, it is time to back up and look at the bigger picture rather than simply "treating" them repeatedly.

If frequent colds and flu are causing the Eustachian tubes to swell, follow the guidelines given in the previous chapter. In the vast majority of cases, chronic Eustachian tube swelling can be traced to allergies and hypersensitivities to casein—the protein found in milk and dairy products.* It has been shown that complete elimination of all traces of casein from the diet prevents over 90% of recurrent otitis media in children. Of the remaining 10%, wheat (gluten) causes about half, and most of the rest are caused by other food, environmental or chemical sensitivities.[2]

No parent wants to see his or her child in pain, which is why so many rush to the pediatrician right away. However, several other therapies can be used at the very first sign of ear pain to try to reverse the problem before the it becomes unbearable, including chiropractic adjustment, decongestant nasal spray and the careful use of a heating pad. Although none of these treatments address the underlying *cause* of chronic ear infections (chronic swelling of the Eustachian tubes), all are excellent alternatives to antibiotic treatment, which is nearly always counter-productive.

Supportive Alternatives

Chiropractic adjustments, especially of the upper cervical area, have been shown to assist the middle ear in draining. In a study conducted by New York chiropractor Dr. Joan Fallon, 80% of children treated with a series of chiropractic adjustments remained free of ear infections for at least six months following their initial treatment. Another study found that 93% of otitis media episodes improved through chiropractic adjustments, 75% of the cases improving in ten days or less, and 43% with only one or two adjustments.[3]

---

* See Chapter 9: *Allergy and Hypersensitivity,* Chapter 10: *Recurrent Colds and Flu,* Chapter 27: *Elimination/Provocation Diet* and Chapter 30: *Avoiding Unnecessary Antibiotics.*

Next, oxymetazoline hydrochloride nasal spray is one of my favorite conventional medical treatments because it does more than simply suppress symptoms—it promotes drainage. As soon as symptoms first appear, use the nasal spray every twelve hours around the clock (for up to two weeks) in order to allow the Eustachian tubes to remain open consistently enough for any fluids to drain out. Granted, getting a child to cooperate with this can be challenging. After spraying into the nostrils, instruct the child to sniff in hard. For an infant, use only 1–2 drops of the pediatric strength formula.

Finally, I have found that applying a heating pad to the ear usually brings some welcome pain relief. Instruct the child to lie down with the painful ear facing up. Set the heat on low, and place the heating pad gently over the ear for 20–30 minutes, 3–4 times per day. Never allow your child to lie down on a heating pad; not only are they at risk for getting burned, but in this position gravity may cause swelling—the opposite of the desired effect.

CHAPTER 12

Recurrent Headaches

If we doctors threw all our medicines into the sea,
it would be that much better for our patients,
and that much worse for the fishes.

~ Oliver Wendell Holmes, MD
(American professor, lecturer and author, 1809–1894)

Common Versus "Normal"

Recurrent, painful, life-altering headaches are so *exceedingly* common, many people have come to think of them as "normal." If you yourself don't suffer from at least the occasional episode, chances are you know several people who do. This chapter describes some very effective holistic remedies for both short and long-term relief. Before going any further, it is important to identify the difference between *acute* headaches and *chronic* headaches.

Acute headaches are those occasional short term headaches most people experience from time to time. The term "acute" has nothing to do with the severity of the headache pain, but instead refers to factors relating to sudden onset and short duration. The causes of acute headaches tend to be easily identified, such as accompanying the onset of a viral illness like a cold or the flu. Most acute headaches simply resolve on their own within a short period of time or, if desired, can often be successfully relieved with pain medications and/or topical decongestants.

Chronic headaches, on the other hand, are those that interfere with your life on a regular basis. The term "chronic" refers to headaches that are recurrent or of a longer duration. Unlike acute headaches, the causes of chronic headaches are more difficult to identify. Chronic headaches are also much more challenging to control with conventional medical approaches. Although the focus of this chapter will be on chronic headaches, keep in mind that the solutions offered can be helpful in resolving most acute headaches as well.

While there are dozens of types of chronic headaches, this chapter will describe the two main categories that make up over 99% of them: *muscle tension* (musculoskeletal) and *vascular*. The remaining less than 1% of chronic headaches are extremely rare and can be due to causes such as autoimmune conditions, tumors and surgically correctable conditions. Given these odds, chances are well in your favor that by following the advice in this chapter, your chronic headaches *can* be permanently resolved.

Tension Headaches

The first and most common of the two types of chronic headaches is the muscle tension headache. Often simply called a "tension headache," this type of headache is significantly painful, yet dull and non-throbbing. The sensation can be described as pressure or tightness in the forehead, sides or back of the head, or some will simply say it hurts "all over."

Even most so-called "sinus headaches" are, at their base, muscle tension headaches. With a sinus headache, the tension in the masseter (jaw) muscle blocks the pterygoid plexus venous return from the sinuses, causing the congestion which then leads to the headache.[1] Headaches due to eyestrain and temperomandibular joint dysfunction (TMJ or TMJD) also fall in the category of muscle tension headaches. Eyestrain headaches occur from unconscious continual movement by the head trying to maintain the highest level of focus, and TMJ headaches occur from chronic muscle tension within the jaw.

Since the underlying cause of muscle tension headaches is the accumulation of stored stress-effect in the hypothalamus (leading to bracing), the only lasting solution for reversing this process once and for all involves following the guidelines of the 3LS Wellness lifestyle.

Vascular Headaches

The second most common type of chronic headache is the vascular headache, which are identifiable by the presence of certain defining characteristics. First, all vascular headaches cause a sharper, *throbbing* pain, unlike the dull or steady pain that is characteristic of muscle tension headaches. If you can count every heartbeat with the throbbing pain in your head, it is classified as a vascular headache. If you cannot, it is a muscle tension headache.

Another defining feature of vascular headaches is that they tend to cause pain on only one side of the head at a time. Since the enervation of the head is divided exactly down the middle, it would be highly unusual for any vascular headache to affect both the right and left sides of the head at the same time. You may have a left-sided vascular headache one week and a right-sided one the next, but only coincidentally could you have both sides throbbing in pain at the same time. Rare exceptions to this rule include the small percentage of vascular headaches that have underlying autoimmune or allergic causation.

The basic mechanism of all vascular headaches involves a loss of vascular tone in the tiny muscles along the walls of the arteries in the head, allowing them to swell with each tiny surge of blood flow. Since there is little room for swelling in the head, a pulse of pain is experienced with each beat of the heart. The fact that these arteries are swelling indicates an underlying dysautonomia because the autonomic nervous system regulates the vascular tone of the arteries. The only way to resolve this problem is to reverse the underlying dysautonomia.*

Migraine Headaches

Migraine, a specific type of vascular headache, is generally over-diagnosed. While it is true that all migraine headaches are vascular, the reverse is not true. Not all vascular headaches are true migraines. In fact, migraine headaches represent a rather uncommon type of vascular headache. True classical migraines differ from other vascular headaches in that migraines include additional symptoms such as nausea, vomiting, sensitivity to

---

* For an in-depth description of dysautonomia, see *The Role of Stress in LGS* in Chapter 7: *Leaky Gut Syndrome*. The solution is a Wellness lifestyle. To understand *why* Wellness works to reverse chronic dis-ease, see Section II: *Precursors to Chronic Health Conditions*. To learn *how* to incorporate Wellness into your everyday life, see Section IV: *The 3-Legged Stool (3LS) of Wellness*.

light and/or a phenomenon known as the "aura." The aura refers to a distortion of perception, with symptoms such as visual disturbances, dizziness, confusion, hypersensitivity and/or euphoria. It occurs *prior* to the onset of the throbbing pain, generally lasting from twenty minutes to an hour. About 15–20% of migraine sufferers experience these and other aura symptoms, which are sometimes mistaken for separate conditions.[2]

Many physicians are in the habit of diagnosing any severe headache as a "migraine." This generally serves to impress the patient that the doctor is validating the pain, since most people associate the word "migraine" with "severe." In fact, a muscle tension headache is often no less severe than a vascular headache.

When people repeatedly treat their headaches with pain-relieving medications, eventually the medications themselves can perpetuate the cycle by causing "rebound headaches." Caffeine is a common ingredient in many over-the-counter migraine medications because it has the effect of constricting blood vessels. While sometimes helpful for an acute episode of pain, repeated caffeine intake can ironically contribute to the vicious cycle of repeated headache episodes over the long run because headache is one of the most common symptoms of caffeine withdrawal.[3]

Breaking the Vicious Cycle

People who suffer frequent headaches often eventually end up with a combination of both muscle tension and vascular components. What begins as a vascular headache can lead to a muscle tension headache in response to the pain you experience from it, and vice versa. The following are some of my favorite holistic remedies, all of which can be safely tried at home and none of which require a prescription. Personal experience of results speaks much louder than words!

As its name suggests, muscle tension headaches are brought on by chronic muscle tension of the head, neck and shoulder muscles and as such, respond quickly to any action that serves to lessen the tension in these areas. If your muscles are chronically tense (bracing), you are likely deficient in magnesium. While working toward correcting the deficiency, heat combined with gentle massage to the shoulder, neck and jaw muscles will often provide relief during a painful episode. (Note: Heat should never be applied to the head for vascular headaches.)

Between headache episodes, stretching and gentle exercises will help relieve some of the muscle tightness that precipitates tension headaches. More comprehensive therapies such as chiropractic adjustments, deep-tissue therapeutic massages, Rolfing, Hellerwork and cranial osteopathy are also extremely helpful preventives.[4] In my opinion, all therapies listed in this paragraph are best utilized when you are not actively experiencing headache pain.

On the other hand, self-hypnosis, deep breathing exercises, acupuncture, acupressure and/or the Emotional Freedom Technique (EFT, a procedure related to acupuncture that involves simple tapping along specific meridian points) all have the potential for both relieving current pain *and* preventing future episodes of both types of headache. In fact, the more pain you are in, the more successful things like self-hypnosis and EFT can be at relieving it.

In addition, I frequently recommend sufferers of any kind of chronic pain address factors such as posture and movement by learning and practicing either the Feldenkrais Method or the Alexander Technique (one or the other, not both). Each of these involve learning how to be more aware of your posture and movement in everyday activities such as standing, sitting and lying, so as to regain your natural grace, reduce tension and promote better health.

What follows next is a simple holistic remedy for immediate relief of vascular headache pain involving nothing but a sink full of hot water.

The "Hot Arms Trick"

It is well known that vascular headache sufferers tend to have cold hands and feet, a sign of decreased circulation throughout the body. Although circulation is actually reduced over the entire skin's surface, hands and feet are the most affected since they are farthest from the heart. Sophisticated biofeedback research has demonstrated that cold extremities are especially noticeable both prior to onset and during the headache episodes. This serves as convincing evidence that the vascular headache sufferer is operating in chronic fight-or-flight (FOF) mode.

Based on the knowledge that when hand/foot blood vessels constrict, cerebral (brain) blood vessels dilate (and vice versa), my favorite remedy for a vascular headache is an immediate biofeedback tool that I like to call the "Hot Arms Trick." The Hot Arms Trick is safe, costs nothing, works as quickly as IV morphine and gives you a sense of control over your headaches you wouldn't otherwise have.

Hot Arms Trick

- Run the kitchen sink full of hot water. The water should be just uncomfortably hot—*not* hot enough to burn your skin!
- Submerge your hands and arms up to, and including, the elbows for 10 minutes.
- The trick is to keep the water at the limit of tolerance the whole time. Add more hot water as it cools.
- Within 10 minutes, most vascular headaches will be gone.

Despite its effectiveness, the Hot Arms Trick could never be considered a *cure* for chronic vascular headaches because it does nothing toward reversing the underlying causes, or toward preventing your next episode. It is, however, a safe and effective alternative treatment. Keep in mind that if you have a combination headache, the Hot Arms Trick will work for the throbbing vascular portion of the headache, but the muscle tension component will likely remain.

Once you have successfully used this method a few times, you can experiment with accomplishing the same result by using imagery, *without* the sink of hot water. Sitting quietly away from distractions, take a few slow, deep breaths, and just imagine exactly how it felt when you submerged your hands and arms in the hot water. With practice, you will find that this visualization exercise will often stop the headache just as effectively. If you are among the 20% who experience an aura, begin the imagery as soon as the aura appears and you will have a good chance of short-circuiting the upcoming onset of pain.

The power of the mind to affect the body cannot be understated. In a lecture given by C. Norman Shealy, MD, PhD, I learned that anything that distracts the sufferer from focusing on pain is likely to provide some measure of relief. To demonstrate this point, try the following experiment. During a painful headache episode, get into the most relaxed state possible. Now, give the headache a flavor. Allow that flavor to become as real as possible in your mind. Next, give the headache a sound. Slowly, one by one, continue giving the headache characteristics such as shape, color, length, odor, age, sex, weight, cost, frequency and so forth. Take your time imagining each characteristic, fully feeling it as you go along. Most headaches will be gone before imagining the tenth characteristic.

Distracting the mind from its current focus is the principle that so often works when someone is about to faint. Many people are rushed to the hospital for fainting, only to be told after spending thousands of dollars on tests that they are perfectly fine. In most cases, if you can get your mind off the fainting, you will not actually faint. This is the reason for placing ammonia perles ("smelling salts") under the nose. They smell so shockingly bad that you stop focusing inwardly (the cause of the fainting) and are forced to focus outwardly (the solution to the fainting). Of course, if your fainting really is due to a valid physiological mechanism, it may not be prevented by this method.

Holistic Headache Solutions

As with all chronic conditions, the real solution to headaches lies in going beyond the mindset of simply treating symptoms, including the holistic treatments offered in this chapter. True resolution will only be achieved when you address the causative mechanisms. Otherwise, although you may have found effective ways to alleviate each headache episode, you have done nothing to prevent yourself from experiencing the next.

For the long-term resolution of chronic headaches, all of the factors addressed in Section II of this book come into play. First, hypothalamic overload of stored stress-effect (fight or flight) must be acknowledged and understood. Second, most sufferers also have leaky gut syndrome (LGS), allowing certain triggering peptides to get into the bloodstream. Third, Candida-related syndrome (C-RS) is often present, a condition that cannot exist aside from LGS.

All of these causative factors can be addressed by practicing the 3LS Wellness guidelines outlined in Section IV of this book. When so doing, I have found that chronic muscle tension headaches tend to resolve in about 3–6 months and chronic vascular headaches in about 6–12 months. If that seems like a long time to wait, let me assure you that chronic headaches will *never* be resolved by simply taking pills (symptom suppression)!

CHAPTER 13

Endocrine Disorders

You desire to know the art of living, my friend?
It is contained in one phrase: make use of suffering.

~ Henri-Frederic Amiel
(Swiss philosopher, poet and critic, 1821–1881)

The Glandular Network

As recently as a half century ago, it was widely believed that the body, mind and spirit were three separate entities. The physician took care of the body, the psychiatrist took care of the mind and the minister (or rabbi, priest, etc.) took care of the spirit. Each territory was jealously guarded. Finally, more and more people are coming to the understanding that everything is connected. Every single aspect of an individual (physical, mental or spiritual) influences every other single aspect. Even more so than with any of the other chronic conditions covered in this section, endocrine disorders must be addressed by seeing the patient as a *whole*.

The endocrine system consists of all the hormone-secreting glands throughout the body. These include the pituitary, thyroid, parathyroids, adrenals, pancreas, pineal, thymus, appendix, testes, ovaries, breasts and the entire lymphatic system. The hypothalamus is considered a neuroendocrine gland. The glandular network operates very much like a spider web—you cannot touch one strand without the effect reverberating throughout the entire web, nor can you break a strand without weakening the entire web.[1]

The pituitary gland was long considered the "master gland" of the body because it controls so many other endocrine glands including the thyroid, breasts, ovaries, testicles, pancreas and adrenals. However, it is now known that the cortex of the brain is the head honcho and the pituitary is simply responding to the orders given by the hypothalamus. As an analogy, if the cortex were considered God (supreme being) and the hypothalamus were considered the president (highest rank in charge), the pituitary would be the chief of staff and the thyroid the governor.

The pituitary gland is made up of two lobes (posterior and anterior) in intimate association with one another. Embryologically, the posterior lobe actually buds and develops off the brain tissue (specifically, the hypothalamus), and the anterior lobe buds and develops off the body tissue (in the thyroid area). Eventually, these two lobes mate at their permanent location in the brain—a *literal* meeting of the body and the mind.

The anterior lobe of the pituitary serves as the body's interface with the brain. This lobe maintains a constant feedback loop of communication with every other endocrine gland in the body. This is crucial because the pituitary's job is to constantly regulate how much of each individual hormonal substance is needed from each individual endocrine gland at any particular point in time. This feedback loop tends to regulate itself (homeostasis) unless aberrant input from an overburdened hypothalamus instructs it to react differently (homeodynamics).[2]

Women are particularly vulnerable when hormonal imbalances occur because the female reproductive organs are all hormonally connected. Common conditions resulting from female hormonal imbalance include fibrocystic breast disease, thyroid disorders, recurrent ovarian cysts, endometriosis, pelvic pain, premenstrual syndrome (PMS), abnormal menstrual bleeding patterns, acne, infertility, hirsutism (abnormal body hair), recurrent bladder infections, chronic vaginitis, painful intercourse and low libido.

Of course, men are not immune to endocrine disturbances either. In males, common problems include prostate disorders, testicular cancers, thyroid disorders and sexual dysfunction (such as impotence and low libido). Whether you are male or female, conventional medicine has only symptom suppressive treatments to offer for all of these increasingly common and intensely frustrating conditions. This chapter will focus on fibrocystic breast disease and thyroid disorders. However, since nearly *all* glandular disorders follow the same patterns, the very same suggestions offered here can be successfully applied to improve or resolve *any* endocrine disorder.

Fibrocystic Breast Disease

Fibrocystic breast disease (FBD) is an extremely common benign (non-cancerous) condition of painful lumps in the breasts that respond to monthly hormonal cycles. These lumps can be fibrous (dense, scar-like tissue) and/or cystic (fluid-filled sacs)—thus the term "fibrocystic." FBD can almost always be resolved with a combination of lifestyle modifications along with specific supplements.

There is currently some controversy over whether caffeine is truly a major contributing factor to FBD. In my experience, caffeine has both a direct toxic effect as well as effects that are somewhat immunological in nature. In genetically susceptible women, even the slightest trace of caffeine seems to trigger something in the immune system that perpetuates the lumps and discomfort. The only way to find out whether caffeine plays a significant role for you is to experiment with a period of total elimination. Do some research before beginning, because when caffeine is *naturally* present in a food or drink (such as with chocolate and black tea), chances are it won't be listed on the label. Keep in mind that even "decaffeinated" products such as coffee and tea still have traces of caffeine.

Over a century ago, a highly concentrated iodine solution called Lugol's was used to treat certain thyroid conditions (such as goiter) and as a surgical prep for thyroidectomy in order to prevent "thyroid storm"—a potentially deadly condition. It was serendipitously discovered that patients who also had FBD began reporting significant improvement in their fibrocystic lesions and pain. Later, in a study involving over seven hundred patients, 95% experienced complete resolution of FBD within one year of taking Lugol's solution alone.[3] Lugol's solution, as well as a convenient tablet form called Iodoral, are available without a prescription.

According to the book, *Iodine, Why You Need It, Why You Can't Live Without It* by David Brownstein, MD, iodine deficiency is far more common in the population than people recognize. Brownstein's research shows that in some individuals, iodine deficiency alone may be one of the *main factors* in endocrine disorders as well as certain cancers, heart disease, multiple sclerosis, certain autoimmune disorders and more.[4] To lessen any possibility of harm, iodine supplementation at pharmacological doses is best done under the supervision of a practitioner experienced with the very latest research in this realm.

While eliminating caffeine and supplementing with iodine, faster and better results can be obtained by taking at least 800 IU of natural vitamin E (mixed tocopherols) daily. This is due to the fact that breast tissue contains a significant proportion of fatty tissue (depending on your age and weight), and vitamin E is a fat-soluble antioxidant.

And finally, in addition to following the 3LS Wellness guidelines given in Section IV of this book, I find a low-fat, high-fiber diet of Whole Foods universally helpful for women with FBD. Initial benefits from this combination of caffeine elimination, iodine and vitamin E supplementation, and lifestyle modifications will generally be obvious within about three months.

Hyperthyroidism and Graves'

Hyperthyroidism (overactive thyroid), of which Graves' disease (an autoimmune version) is just one manifestation, was one of the first common forms of thyroid pathology definitively linked to stress.[5] It is no wonder, since the hypothalamus controls pituitary function, and the thyroid is directly involved in the pituitary feedback loop.

Secreted by the pituitary gland, thyroid stimulating hormone (TSH) does exactly as its name suggests—it stimulates the thyroid to produce more thyroid hormone. When the TSH is high, the thyroid is under-functioning and you are diagnosed as *hypo*thyroid. The message the pituitary is sending to the thyroid is "more, more!" When the TSH is low, the thyroid is over-functioning and you are diagnosed as *hyper*thyroid. The message the pituitary is sending to the thyroid is "too much already!"

Actually, Graves' is not a primary disease of the thyroid. Graves' occurs when the hypothalamus, chronically overwhelmed by stress-effect storage, tries to compensate by telling the pituitary to produce more TSH (turning up the metabolism). Blood work showing an initial high TSH (hypothyroid) phase should be viewed as a universal sign of impending Graves', however this warning generally goes unheard. If the high TSH is not successfully recognized and reversed in time, the thyroid eventually burns out and the TSH goes from too high to too low. By the time an individual has the classic symptoms of Graves', the pituitary portion of the hypothalamic cascade is already exhausted.

Conventional options for Graves' disease include either surgical removal of the thyroid gland or burning it out with radioactive iodine (RAI). Complications of surgery include the risks of accidental damage or removal of the parathyroid glands (causing a major life-long upset of the body's calcium balance with serious consequences) and/or damage to the laryngeal nerve (resulting in temporary or permanent loss of normal speech function). Complications of RAI include very minor risks of cancer and very major risks of sudden or eventual hypothyroidism.

Until or unless the accumulated stress-effect storage in the hypothalamus is discharged, the physiological pathology will continue to progress long after the thyroid has been destroyed or removed. Given this fact, how can either surgery or RAI be considered a *cure* for thyroid dysfunction by any standard?

Hypothyroidism and Hashimoto's

Unless brought about through thyroidectomy or RAI treatment, hypothyroidism (under-active thyroid) is now known to be frequently caused by so many years of overstimulation by the pituitary that the thyroid finally becomes worn out. The allopathic monopoly, presently calling all the shots in this country, focuses entirely on treating this condition only *after* it is too late to reverse the causes.[6]

In medical school, we were taught that the treatment of hypothyroidism with oral thyroid hormone medication was one of the greatest successes in allopathic medicine—on par with treating diabetes with insulin. Granted, once things have progressed to that point, it is true that oral hormone replacement is still the best approach and does, indeed, result in great benefits for the patient. However, pharmaceuticals will never be as smart as nature.

The normal, healthy thyroid makes a different amount, and type, of thyroid hormone each day. Thyroid pills, on the other hand, often provide too much or too little thyroid hormone on any given day. In a healthy individual, the hypothalamus analyzes how much thyroid hormone is needed, based on ever-changing physical, emotional and environmental influences, and reports back to the pituitary. The pituitary then produces a certain amount of TSH telling the thyroid how much thyroid hormone to produce.

No matter how accurate the physician may try to be, no pill can do as well as a healthy, self-regulating human system can. The best any physician can do is figure out an average dose and prescribe that same dose every day, adjusting it periodically according to how the patient is faring. With thyroid-replacement medication, a patient is, in effect, getting the *wrong* thyroid dose nearly every day. The rest of the endocrine glands in the "web" must then accommodate to this discrepancy, making the entire bodymind system a little less competent, and making the individual much more susceptible to all forms of acute and chronic conditions.

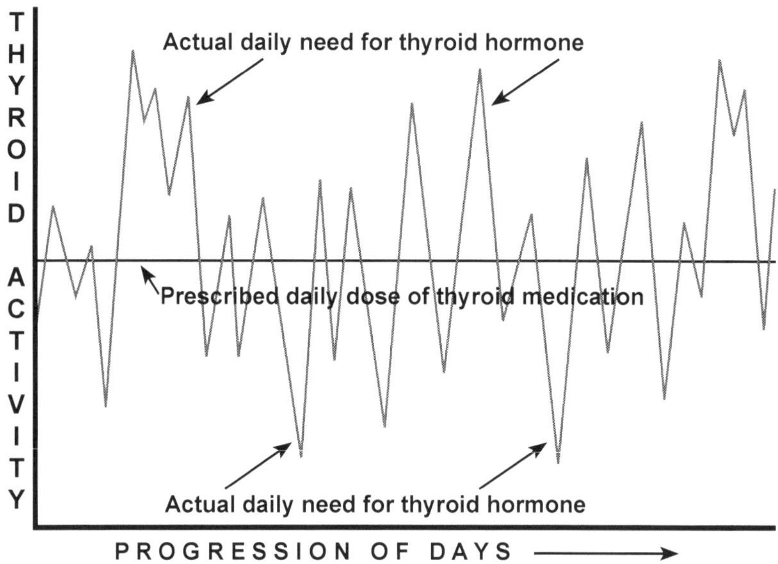

Relative Need of Thyroid Hormone

Hashimoto's disease is one possible version of hypothyroidism. Like Graves', Hashimoto's involves an autoimmune process, meaning the immune system mistakenly begins attacking the body's own tissues. Autoimmune attacks are very specific. In one person the attack may be against the thyroid, in another person the attack may be the joints, connective tissues, blood elements, etc. In my opinion, at least 90% of all autoimmunity begins with leaky gut syndrome (LGS).

Obviously missing from this picture is that, with the proper information, the thyroid gland could have been prevented from failing in the first place. Holistic-minded physicians look for signs of hypothalamic overstimulation years before impending failure, and encourage the patient to take steps toward prevention. With those for whom it's already too late, discharging the hypothalamic burden is just as important.

The Spider Web Analogy

Remember that spider web analogy given at the beginning of this chapter? It is important because no matter which specific manifestation(s) of endocrine dysfunction you may be experiencing symptomatically, the entire glandular system is being affected *whether you realize it or not*. Therefore, by resolving (reversing the causes) of any one glandular disorder, the entire network will benefit and over-all health will be greatly improved.

As described in Chapters 5 and 6, the physical, chemical, environmental, psychosocial and spiritual load modern humans are struggling to cope with has created an overwhelming stress-effect burden and forced the hypothalamus to try to function in ways for which it was never designed. One of the unexpected consequences of the resulting alteration of our immune system reserves is leaky gut syndrome (LGS) and Candida-related syndrome (C-RS). The toxic by-products of Candida's active fungal phase have a direct effect on the endocrine system—especially in women.

The good news is that the resolution of endocrine disorders or at the very least, impressive health benefits, can be obtained by following the 3LS Wellness guidelines in this book. Within 6–12 months of diligent practice, most endocrine disorders will be either resolved or greatly improved, because every single organ system in the bodymind is influenced by the hypothalamus through its direct influence on the pituitary.

CHAPTER 14

Vascular Disorders

The greater the ignorance, the greater the dogmatism.

~ Sir William Osler, MD
(Canadian physician, historian and author, 1849–1919)

What Are "Vascular Disorders"?

The vascular system refers to the network of blood vessels (arteries, veins, capillaries and lymphoid system) that carry blood and fluids throughout the body. Vascular disorders, therefore, refer to conditions that affect this circulatory system such as heart attacks, strokes and loss of circulation to the legs. These are among the most deadly, expensive and devastating disorders in our society—they are also among the least likely to be successfully managed by the allopathic treatment philosophy and, as this chapter will demonstrate, a good example of the dangers inherent in allowing one solitary healing paradigm to monopolize our thinking.

Blood pressure abnormalities often precede vascular events. "Blood pressure" refers to the amount of force (or pressure) the blood is exerting in the walls of the arteries. A blood pressure readings involve two numbers. The first number (systolic) represents the amount of pressure when the heart *beats*, and the second number (diastolic) represents the amount of pressure when the heart is *at rest*—between beats. Previous American Heart Association guidelines defined a "normal" reading as anything below 140/90 mm Hg (millimeters of mercury). However, more recent guidelines have reduced those numbers and today, anything above 120/80 is considered abnormal.[1] Of course, many factors (including anxiety over a visit to the doctor) can temporarily affect blood pressure, so be sure to take the average of several readings and test in a relaxed setting if possible.

High blood pressure is often called "the silent killer" because the outward signs typically don't even *begin* to appear until blood pressure has gone uncontrolled (high) for about fifteen years. Signs and symptoms of hypertension might include chest pain, swelling in the ankles, coldness or loss of strength in an extremity, shortness of breath with exertion or while lying down at night, headaches, a gradually increasing resting heart rate, remarkable heart rate increases with the simplest exertion, cramps in the legs when walking (with progressively shorter distances), fluid accumulation in the abdomen (as evidenced by looking pregnant), changes in bowel habits due to poor circulation in the gut, and visual changes necessitating a visit to the ophthalmologist.

Once symptoms finally become apparent, it can take an average of five additional years for totally uncontrolled hypertension to cause things like coronary heart disease, heart attacks, strokes, atherosclerosis, peripheral vascular disease, kidney damage or enlargement of the heart due to congestive heart failure.

Low blood pressure (hypotension) before middle age is also a red flag. Hypotension is a clear warning sign that the system already has insufficient reserves for keeping blood pressure within normal range. People with low blood pressure early in life are at higher risk of developing high blood pressure later in life, unless steps are taken to prevent its progression. In most cases, both hypertension and hypotension are simply two stages of the same process—dysautonomia.

Coronary heart disease (also called coronary artery disease and ischemic heart disease) is the most common type of heart disease in the United States and a leading cause of death in both men *and* women. This disease involves a progressive build up of plaque (comprised of various substances circulating in the blood such as cholesterol, calcium, cellular waste and inflammatory byproducts) inside the coronary arteries. This built-up plaque eventually begins to obstruct the flow of oxygen-rich blood to the heart to a greater or lesser degree.

Conventional medical treatment options for coronary heart disease include cholesterol lowering medications, blood thinners (aspirin, etc.), pain medications for angina (chest pain), and surgical procedures such as cardiac catheterization, placement of stents and coronary bypass surgery. Unless the patient is significantly overweight, the condition is generally blamed on genetics and salt avoidance is often the only lifestyle suggestion emphasized.

The Pritikin/Ornish Program

In the 1950s, Dr. Nathan Pritikin (not an MD) was diagnosed with advanced coronary heart disease at a very young age. He embarked on a journey of discovery about world cultures that enjoyed the lowest incidence of heart disease. Based on his research findings, he began exercising regularly, practicing relaxation techniques and eating a diet consisting of less than 10% of total calories from fat. So amazed was he at the rapidity of his improvement, he named this protocol the "Pritikin Program" and made it his life's work to help others achieve the same results.[2]

Unfortunately, too many cardiac surgeons had already been trained to believe that lifestyle had little or nothing to do with chronic disease, so Pritikin was called a fraud by the medical establishment. Even after his program was featured twice on CBS' *60 Minutes* in the late 1970s as being routinely successful, conventional medicine refused to acknowledge this alternative to their now practically routine approach of coronary bypass surgery. Perhaps if this plan had been available "by prescription only," a different story could be told.

The 10% fat diet works by forcing the body to scavenge for stored fat in order to make vital hormones. One of the places the body takes this fat from is the interior walls of the arteries. What Pritikin failed to understand, however, is that once the stored fat is used up and the atherosclerotic condition has been reversed (about a year or two, depending on how closely the plan is followed), dietary fat intake *must* be increased to 15% for lifetime maintenance. Pritikin stayed on the 10% diet too long, and ended up dying of cancer about forty years later. However, his autopsy revealed the coronary arteries of a 16-year old.

In the early 1980s, Dean Ornish, MD slightly revised the Pritikin Program and renamed it "Dr. Dean Ornish's Program for Reversing Heart Disease." In his *New York Times* best-selling book by that name, his research documented that candidates for coronary bypass surgery could be given a choice between surgery and the Pritikin/Ornish Program. Of his patients who chose the lifestyle approach, 90% became asymptomatic within one month. Ornish's research was published in the *Journal of the American Medical Association (JAMA)*, one of the most conservative medical journals in the United States.[3]

EDTA Chelation Therapy

Around 1976–77, my own mother came to me (a.k.a. "my son, the doctor") complaining of transient ischemic attacks (TIAs). After finding an abnormal sound over one of her carotid arteries, I sent her for a routine arteriogram in preparation for surgery (still the standard treatment to this day). Sadly, the injection of the x-ray dye into her artery caused her to have a stroke (not an uncommon complication). This unfortunate event made it impossible to finish the arteriogram or do the surgery.

A year later, while mostly recovered from the stroke, she continued to suffer TIAs. Having had enough of my advice, she took matters into her own hands and went to Columbus, Ohio for EDTA (ethylene diamine tetra-acetic acid) chelation therapy, a major complementary approach to vascular insufficiency. I never forgot how much the treatments did for her. She not only got rid of her TIAs, she also looked and acted ten years younger. The results were so dramatic, it would have been dishonest of me to continue to tell my patients that surgery was their only option. Keep in mind that chelating physicians are trained to counsel patients that a healthy lifestyle alongside the EDTA chelation therapy is the combination that brings results.

EDTA chelation (pronounced "key-lay-shun") therapy is an outpatient procedure involving intravenous transfusions of chelating agents. Taking about three and a half hours to perform, the chelating agents draw out and bind with heavy metals and toxic metabolic wastes in the bloodstream, allowing them to be eliminated by the body. In addition, the chelating agents remove the calcium content of plaque and toxic ions from arterial walls, restoring circulation (and therefore better immune function) to all tissues of the body.[4] Most chelating physicians recommend 20–30 sessions for optimal results.

In the early 1980s, Elmer Cranton, MD, author of *Bypassing Bypass*, reported that EDTA chelation therapy seemed to work by reversing free radical pathology.[5] At that time, conventional physicians had never heard of free radicals (or antioxidants) and any such talk was considered quackery. Today, management of free radical reactions is considered a "breakthrough" in orthodox medicine.

After my mother's turnaround, I took the necessary training to be able to incorporate intravenous EDTA chelation therapy into my practice, following the protocol taught by the international training and certification organization for chelation (the American College for Advancement in Medicine). Although I had no vascular symptoms, I decided that my first patient would be myself. Sure enough, I had more energy and a greater sense of well-being for at least a year following the series.

Prior to my EDTA training and certification, I routinely sent an average of five patients per year to the cardiac surgeon. Once I was able to offer this therapy, of all the patients who chose to follow my instructions (including the lifestyle changes) throughout the remainder of my career, only one had to be sent for bypass surgery. The rest (an estimated seventy patients) not only avoided the risk and expense of surgery, but also enjoyed a much higher quality of life than my former post-surgical patients did. Additionally, *all* of my patients with diabetic gangrene (some of which were also heart patients) were able to avoid the debilitating amputation surgeries their conventional physicians were recommending. The only unfortunate downside to this whole experience was the harassment I received by my state medical licensing board.

When I offered EDTA chelation therapy for chronic obstructive vascular disease, my patients enjoyed numerous unexpected side benefits. I saw arthritis improve, diabetes improve, hypertension disappear, chronic rashes clear up, and more. I even saw a very large life-long goiter (enlargement of the thyroid gland) disappear. EDTA is just one of many examples of drugs that have been shown to improve conditions totally unrelated to the ones for which they were first developed.

Off-Label Drug Uses and the FDA

Intravenous EDTA first originated as the standard of treatment for severe lead poisoning in the 1940s. At that time, low-level lead toxicity was considered insignificant, so most people weren't diagnosed until they were finally at death's door. Administering very high doses of EDTA quickly removed enough lead to save the person's life. However, since EDTA is excreted through the kidneys along with the lead, patients occasionally suffered kidney damage from the procedure. Given that the alternative was death, the treatment was still used.

Within the first ten years of its use, people being treated with EDTA for lead intoxication began reporting improvements in their angina, arthritis, hypertension, and other health complaints as an unexpected side benefit. At first, it was assumed that the removal of lead caused the improvement. Subsequently, it was found that the improvements were directly related to the EDTA *itself*, and had little or nothing to do with the lead removal.[6]

Soon it was discovered that much lower doses of EDTA were just as effective for achieving these peripheral vascular benefits without damaging the kidneys. This allowed the development of the international protocol I mentioned earlier. Yet even today, when asked about EDTA by their patients facing surgery, many physicians warn of the terrible risk of kidney damage. This is a great example of how too little information can be a dangerous thing. As a matter of fact, Emanuel Cheraskin, MD, DMD has reported that in *all* cases where EDTA chelation therapy was done according to international protocol, kidney function actually *improved*.

Macular degeneration is an excellent example of a disorder which is almost universally benefitted by EDTA chelation therapy. Macular degeneration is a vascular condition of the retinal blood vessels that begins with blurred vision and can lead to central blindness. All degenerative conditions (of which macular degeneration is a classic one) begin with tissue getting sick and continue to progress when nothing is done about *why* it is getting sick. Long before it dies, it stops functioning. If there is enough tissue still alive, chelation therapy can restore function significantly. Since conventional medicine has no effective treatment for macular degeneration, one can't help but wonder why they don't at least *look* into EDTA. As an official of the FDA was quoted as saying regarding being reluctant to admit they were wrong in persecuting chelating physicians, "That kind of admission would open the gates to quackery."[7]

Patents, Profits and Progress

The FDA's back-and-forth position on EDTA is a perfect example of how money has been calling the shots in our monopolistic disease-care system. For example, the initial side benefits noted with EDTA for heart disease were so undeniable, the Food and Drug Administration (FDA) made a change in the *Physician's Desk Reference* (PDR) in the 1950s to allow it to be legally used for atherosclerosis. (The PDR is the official, annually updated FDA-approved book that lists the latest, most accurate prescription drug information known.) Although approved for atherosclerosis, EDTA failed to gain FDA approval for the many other conditions just described because, at that time, the FDA required every newly discovered application of a drug to be tested as though it were a *new* drug—a process that takes many years and often millions of dollars.

Adding to that obstacle, EDTA had already been on the market so long by the 1950s it could no longer be patented. As with any drug, without a patent, any company that spends all that time and money testing it for potential new applications cannot possibly get their research substantiation money back. Moreover, all their competitors would be free to produce the drug for any new application as soon as it was approved by the FDA. As a consequence, the listing about EDTA being an effective treatment for atherosclerosis was removed from the PDR that same decade.

Thankfully, there is one important area in which our health-care system has made an intelligent change. About twenty years ago, the FDA finally ruled that any drug approved for one purpose could be used for any other "off label" purpose subsequently discovered—as long as it was prescribed by a licensed physician. For example, Aminophylline, first used internally for asthma, has been found to smooth out the cellulite (dimpled fat) in women's thighs when used topically. Heparin, a standard drug used to prevent clotting when used intravenously, has been found to be a potent anticancer drug when used orally. Dilantin, used for many years to control epileptic seizures, is now known to be effective for a whole range of serious disorders.[8] Minoxidil, first used orally to control high blood pressure, is now used topically for hair loss.

There are numerous other examples. Perhaps one of the most notable and promising recent ones is low dose Naltrexone (LDN). Naltrexone was originally approved by the FDA in 1984 in a 50 mg dose to help heroin and opiate addicts overcome their addictions by blocking the receptors, and thus the effects, of these drugs. The following year, it was discovered that a much lower dose (1.5–4.5 mg/day taken at bedtime) benefitted people with AIDS, multiple sclerosis, cancer, autism, autoimmune disease and more. This "off label" use of Naltrexone acts as a biomedical treatment, enhancing and improving the body's own immune system by causing an increase in beta-endorphin levels.[9]

"To a Hammer, Everything Looks Like a Nail!"

Prior to the FDA's new ruling, physicians from all over the world had proven EDTA chelation therapy to be an extremely effective treatment for chronic vascular diseases. Yet here in the United States, the allopathic monopoly had already tasted how lucrative bypass surgery was. The AMA, viewing EDTA chelation (a relatively inexpensive treatment—averaging $3,000) as a financial threat to cardiac surgeons and hospitals, began covertly attacking physicians like myself who offered it to their patients. Then in 1994, the Kentucky medical licensing board made it their primary goal to eliminate the option of EDTA chelation for its citizens. As of this writing, they have succeeded in doing so. Several other states have also targeted this particular holistic therapy with the intention of eradicating it.

Medicare has been successfully sued for denying coverage for EDTA chelation therapy. However, the government did an "end run" to prevent anyone using this ruling as a precedent. The ruling stated that each case would have to be pursued through the courts "on an individual basis." Given that it costs more to pursue it this way than it would cost to just pay for the chelation out of pocket, the only cases that have been approved by Medicare were the ones in which the patient was angry enough, and wealthy enough, to go through the entire legal process.

If denying heart patients effective alternatives weren't bad enough, denying them the statistics on coronary bypass surgery is even worse. Most patients who go in for this routine procedure are never informed of research showing that the repaired arteries tend to close up faster than they were closing before the procedure. Most experts now agree that only 11% of all coronary bypass operations are either necessary or appropriate.[10] The other 89% of patients would do better with the short-term 10% fat Pritikin/Ornish Program and/or the EDTA chelation therapy as described in this chapter.

During the first thirteen years of my practice, I knew nothing of alternatives to the strictly conventional approach to vascular disease: Confirm the diagnosis and refer the patient to surgery. After all, "To a hammer, everything looks like a nail!" Referring patients to the bypass surgeon was straightforward for me and placed all the responsibility for future consequences on the surgeon. In my opinion, there are too many daunting statistics available about the risks of that approach that there can be no valid excuse for cardiac physicians today who continue to blindly follow it. Safe and effective alternatives for this and the other chronic conditions in this book continue to take a back seat to our country's profit-driven disease-care treatment approach.

I find it interesting that the monopoly that profits so profusely from bypass surgery continues to insist on repeated double-blind studies for EDTA chelation therapy, yet fails to acknowledge there never could be a double-blind study for coronary bypass surgery. In addition, patients suffering from vascular disease are usually so sick that it would be unethical to give large numbers of them placebos just to give the naysayers more proof of the positive results that hundreds of other studies have already shown.

If the Pritikin/Ornish Program could have been patented and had required a prescription upon its discovery, it would surely have made headline news as a breakthrough of major proportions in the treatment of ischemic heart disease. Yet today, with the exception of some of the most progressive insurance companies, the standard being offered patients is *still* bypass surgery. Most insurance companies won't question paying $100,000 for bypass surgery (which frequently has to be repeated), yet they refuse to reimburse physicians an average of $3,000 for EDTA chelation therapy or less than $1,000 for the necessary education and follow-up to counsel patients on diet, exercise and effective relaxation techniques, known in this book as the 3LS of Wellness.[11]

Protocol for Vascular Insufficiency

There are many ways to prevent and reverse vascular disorders. The suggestions given in this chapter will cause a dramatic and rapid improvement in vascular conditions across the board. In nearly all cases, blood pressure will normalize within six months of practicing the 3LS of Wellness outlined in Section IV of this book. In addition, I recommend the following protocol to *anyone* with vascular insufficiency:

Vascular Insufficiency Protocol*

- Omega 3 essential fatty acid (EFA) supplementation (2,000 mg twice a day).
- High doses of antioxidants such as natural vitamin E (400–800 IU per day, mixed tocopherols), esterified vitamin C (1–2 grams twice a day) and beta carotene.[12] It is interesting to note that prior to 1995, our medical system denied the validity of treating vascular disease with high doses of vitamin E, despite recommendations from knowledgeable holistic physicians for over fifty years. Although most medical journals today openly agree with this holistic remedy, many conventional physicians *still* have not included it as a standard of care for the same reasons so many other safe and effective holistic remedies are being ignored—they are not pharmaceuticals and the system has made profit the criteria for deciding what is acceptable and what is not.
- Balanced vitamin B complex (50–100 mg twice a day).
- Ask your chelating physician about getting an intracellular magnesium test. Not only are optimum magnesium levels an effective preventive, but we now know that patients who are given intravenous magnesium right after a heart attack have a 50% higher survival rate.[13]
- Avoid all stimulants (caffeine, nicotine, sugar, etc.).
- Switch from refined table salt to unrefined mineral salt. Unrefined mineral salt (such as "RealSalt") is mined from ancient sea beds containing 70+ trace minerals. With hypertension, the problem isn't the excess sodium in the diet, but the imbalance caused by the trace minerals missing in refined table salt. Taking a crystalline or ionic mineral supplement in addition to switching to unrefined mineral salt would speed up your progress significantly.

If you are taking antihypertensive medication, it is crucial to work closely with your doctor to safely and gradually reduce your medication as you progress. This includes monitoring your own blood pressure

* See Chapter 28: *Intracellular Magnesium* and Chapter 29: *Essential Fatty Acids.*

frequently at home. Failure to adjust medication dosages as your blood pressure normalizes could lead to hypotensive episodes, causing a more immediate risk of a coronary or stroke than the original hypertension did.

If your physician has an open mind, perhaps he or she will be impressed enough by your rapid progress to want to learn more about what you have been up to. As more and more physicians learn from their patients or read books such as this one, every subsequent patient seen by them will reap the benefits.

CHAPTER 15

Brain Chemistry Disorders

Help others to help themselves,
rather than giving that which makes them poor indeed.

~ Edgar Cayce
(Famous psychic and founder of the A.R.E., 1877–1945)

Moody, Depressed and Obsessed

At some point in our lives, most of us have experienced, at least to some degree, one or more of the many types of brain chemistry disorders. Examples include depression, mood swings, anxiety, panic, phobias, obsessions, compulsions and even addictions. If you've been one of the fortunate few who has never experienced at least one of these conditions firsthand, chances are you know several friends or family members who have.

Disorders of brain chemistry may well be the most poorly managed category of chronic health conditions in this country—and it's big business. On television and in magazines, it's almost impossible to avoid the slew of pharmaceutical advertisements about the latest featured drugs designed to treat these frustrating imbalances. Prescription antidepressant and anti-anxiety medications, often the first and/or only option considered by conventional practitioners, are *extremely* lucrative for the medical/pharmaceutical complex.

When I was in medical school, all "mental illness" was thought to be psychological in nature and therefore counseling was thought to be the best solution. Mainstream medicine has since come to understand that mental illness is at least aggravated by a chemical imbalance in the brain and is in *all* cases a combination of chemistry and psychosocial factors. The question is, how does this imbalance come about in the first place?

The typical scenario is as follows: First, a genetically susceptible individual exceeds his or her personal threshold of the total load of environmental stressors. Once this person has "fallen off the edge of the cliff," brain chemistry becomes altered.* The individual is then forced to develop a vast array of coping mechanisms in order to deal with the now-abnormal brain chemistry. Psychological aspects and aberrant behaviors come into play, which *further* aggravate the original brain chemistry imbalance. Eventually, these secondary behaviors can become so habituated, they must also be addressed even after the brain chemistry has been rebalanced.

From the very same causes, one individual may exhibit depression or anger, whereas another individual may, for example, struggle with anxiety, phobias, substance abuse or an eating disorder. In the vast majority of cases, if people were given the correct information, they could re-balance their brain chemistry naturally without the potential risks and side effects of medication. That is not to imply that medications may not be temporarily useful until the implementation of that information can take effect. The necessary education begins with an understanding of the connection between the brain and the gut.

The Gut-Brain Connection

We physicians have known for at least 50–60 years that there is a direct connection between psychological changes and gut pathology. The old assumption was that the psychological factors *caused* the subsequent alterations in the gut. It looks like we may have had it all backwards: Gut pathology is most likely the *cause* of the psychological changes.[1]

The gut plays a far greater role in the body than digestion alone. In fact, it is now known that the intestinal tract is in effect a "second brain" (perhaps even the primary brain as far as hormone production is concerned). Believe it or not, the digestive tract makes more endorphins (feel-good chemicals) than the brain itself. The "brain of the gut" is known as the enteric nervous system. It mirrors the central nervous system and plays a huge role in the production of neurotransmitters. Some common

---

* See "Are You Walking on the Edge?" in Chapter 5: *Modern Medical Interpretation of Stress.*

examples of how we experience this gut-brain interconnection include "gut feelings," "butterflies in the stomach" or feeling nauseous when anxious or excited about something.

For an in-depth scientific understanding of how the health of the gut affects *every* condition of the bodymind, I recommend Dr. Michael Gershon's groundbreaking book, *The Second Brain*.[2] Dr. Gershon is a professor in the department of anatomy and cell biology at Columbia University College of Physicians and Surgeons. He has been researching the gut-brain connection since 1962, and has published more than three hundred papers on this subject.

As detailed in the first two sections of this book, the number and variety of environmental stressors humans must cope with today—including nutritional stressors—far exceeds what we were being exposed to just one hundred years ago. In addition, activation of fight-or-flight reduces the blood supply available to the gut, leading to leaky gut syndrome (LGS), a precursor to a host of chronic conditions.

Nutrition and Mental Health

Nearly all brain chemistry disorders have environmental (including nutritional) factors playing a significant causative role. One study demonstrated that 89% of patients with mental and neurological symptoms, 84% of patients with mood changes and 45% of patients with minimal brain dysfunction (including attention deficit, hyperactivity, dyslexia and learning disabilities) have food allergies and sensitivities as one of their causes. When coupled with the nutritional deficiencies created by eating a refined diet, one can only imagine the effects on brain chemistry.[3]

Research proving the strong connection between nutrition and mental health has been available for decades, yet our country continues to favor its ongoing disease-care approach. In the 1950s, the pioneering work of Abram Hoffer, MD, PhD demonstrated conclusively that nutrients in orthomolecular doses were many times more effective for schizophrenia (the most difficult kind of brain dysfunction to treat) than any drug and were without any of the negative side effects. Seen as a threat to the conventional medical monopoly, the American Psychiatric Association (APA) not only ridiculed his work, but eventually also tried to deny him the right to continue seeing patients.[4]

Hoffer's was but one of a flurry of publications in the 1950s referring to safe alternative solutions to conventional treatment of schizophrenia. Even Nobel Laureate Linus Pauling recognized the validity of Hoffer's discoveries, yet the APA continues to ignore them to this day. Denial and intentional ignorance are generally the pattern when it would prove intensely embarrassing for the establishment to admit they were wrong. According to Pauling, "The APA bears major responsibility for preventing the introduction of a treatment which would have saved millions of patients from the ravages of chronic schizophrenia. Just as the APA was once captured by psychoanalysis, it is now captured by tranquilizers."[5]

In the 1960s, Dr. Alexander Schauss was another pioneer in educating both the professionals in the field and the public about alternative ways to approach brain chemistry disorders. His book, *Diet, Crime and Delinquency,* documented what nutrition expert and author Dr. Carlton Fredericks and biochemical/nutritional pioneer and author Dr. Roger Williams, among many others, had been reporting since the 1940s about the relationships between brain chemistry, nutrition and behavior. He compared various conventional and alternative options with a variety of poorly managed child behavioral problems and delinquency, finding that 51% showed improvement when sugar was eliminated from the diet, and 50% showed improvement when wheat was eliminated. In addition, 45% showed improvement from taking vitamin supplements, as compared to only 1.6% *from all drugs combined.*[6]

The real question is, since this information has been known since 1977, why has it not been the basis for a major effort by the government to either officially substantiate it or trash it, instead of pretending it doesn't exist? Nutritional and other holistic approaches are being hotly resisted by the AMA and Big Pharma as evidenced by the health-care reform battle in Washington over disease-care policy that escalated in 2009.

In 1980, William Philpott, MD published his landmark book entitled *Brain Allergies,* which is a classic in the field.[7] His book clearly showed that many environmental substances can influence brain chemistry. In 1983, Barbara Reed, PhD published a practical manual for the application of a nutritional approach called *Food, Teens and Behavior.*[8] Over a quarter century after these books were published, numerous studies have been conducted by private foundations supporting the conclusion that there are safe and effective alternatives to drugs and counseling. In the meantime, teenage violence and suicide continues to be a national epidemic and conventional medicine remains manically focused on trying to find a better (more lucrative) pill rather than doing something about *why* brain chemistry becomes altered. How much more does it have to cost our country, both financially and in ruined lives, before the conventional establishment gives this well-established research an honest appraisal?

"Stable Criminal Syndrome"

Over fifty years ago, the veterinary medical profession identified a condition whereby a horse would simply go crazy all of a sudden. They termed this "stable criminal syndrome" because the affected horse in the stable would act like a crazed murderer. With no clue as to the cause and no cure for the bizarre condition, these horses had to be put down—a serious problem that cost many horse breeders dearly.

It was finally discovered that once a susceptible horse became deficient in magnesium, a small dose of phosphorus could then trigger the animal into a killing frenzy. Since grain is very high in phosphorus, this unfortunate scenario occurred frequently. Once the cause was finally understood, all the breeder had to do was ensure normal magnesium levels in the animals.

Magnesium is one of the main nutrients removed during the food refining process. Since the percentage of refined foods has steadily increased over the past century, the average person in this country is deficient in magnesium.[9] What makes this even more interesting is that refined foods, especially soft drinks, are very high in phosphorus. Considering the diet of today's average youth, is it any wonder that those most susceptible to the human equivalent of "stable criminal syndrome" are now showing up in our society in ever-increasing numbers?

In 1849, the average soft drink consumption in the United States was one eight-ounce serving per person per year. Within just ten years, that number jumped to five eight-ounce servings per person per year. In 1919, the number rose to 39 servings; in 1949, 87 servings; and in 1969, 200 servings. By 1976, that number jumped to 493 servings per person per year then by 2002, rose to a whopping 216 *liters*, which is the equivalent of 904 eight-ounce servings per person per year![10] We can no longer afford to assume our country's increased soft drink consumption has nothing to do with the increased prevalence of mental and behavioral disorders.

In children and teenagers (who happen to be the biggest soda drinkers), nutritional deficiencies tend to manifest as various behavioral issues, learning problems and attention deficit disorders. Adults, having a little more maturity and self-control, instead exhibit panic attacks, free floating anxiety and depression, among others. Both children and adults with nutritional deficiencies typically show increased aggressive tendencies. While numerous books have been written on this subject, the facts are swept under the rug in favor of pharmaceutical treatments.

Strong reasons make strong actions.

~ William Shakespeare (1564–1616)

From Drugs to Doing What *Works*

Mental and behavioral problems will continue to increase in our society until the causes are addressed. Presently, the push is toward more law enforcement and harsher punishments for crimes committed by children and teenagers. But is the threat of incarceration an intelligent solution, considering that when brain chemistry is altered there are no thoughts of consequences? Most of the answers are right in front of us, and my hope is that people will begin to see these answers once they decide they have finally suffered enough.

Treating brain chemistry disorders with pharmaceuticals may temporarily manage symptoms, but does nothing to address *why* the imbalance occurred in the first place. This goes back to the critical difference between a treatment and a cure, described in Chapter 1. Until or unless the original causes of mental illness are addressed, the need for conventional treatments can be expected to continue indefinitely. In addition to the high cost and relative ineffectiveness of these drugs, they *all* have negative side effects. Many are even seriously addictive.

The most effective and comprehensive long-term approach to reversing brain chemistry disorders involves taking discharging the hypothalamic overload and healing leaky gut syndrome by practicing the 3LS of Wellness described in Section IV of this book. The quickest and most effective short-term approach is proper nutrition. I have seen the amazing results of altering the diets of my patients with brain chemistry imbalances such as delinquency, learning disabilities, autism, behavior problems, hyperactivity and more.[11] When dietary changes are done right, improvements in behavior are dramatic and immediate. We *know* what to do and we know how to do it, but, again, this type of information is rarely provided by conventional physicians because their paradigm is based on treatments, not cures.

Another advantage of natural approaches that work is that the patient (and the parents) no longer feel the onus of there being "something wrong with me (or my child)." The child starts to think more clearly and function better, and comes to realize he or she does not have to live forever feeling "different," taking medication and seeing a therapist. For children, who want desperately to conform to their peers, this can make a world of difference.

The best way to demonstrate the relationship between nutrition and mental health is to experience it for yourself. Don't talk yourself out of modifying your diet (or your child's) with the old excuse, "If it is so great, why isn't everybody doing it?" or "Why hasn't my doctor told me about it?" *Why* indeed![12] By applying the information in this book, you can experience firsthand the amazing improvements that can be had with the proper diligence and effort. In most cases, the benefits will start to become obvious within the first two weeks.

CHAPTER 16

Arthritic Disorders

There are only two ways to live your life.
One is as though nothing is a miracle.
The other is as though everything is a miracle.

~ Albert Einstein
(Father of modern physics, 1879–1955)

Several Different Types: One Common Cause

The term "arthritis" refers to an inflammatory condition of the joints that can be either traumatic, infective or autoimmune in origin. Some of the most common types of arthritis include rheumatoid arthritis, osteoarthritis, fibromyalgia syndrome (FMS), tendonitis, bursitis and gout. Basically, *any* connective tissue inflammatory condition belongs under the "arthritic disorders" umbrella.

Conventional medicine has come up with a variety of names for these painful and degenerative conditions. Doctors can describe what you might expect from the particular type with which they label you, but can do little to manage or alter the course of this disease. They can attempt to treat the discomfort, but can offer no cures. Many of the medications they prescribe have potentially serious long-term side effects, and *none* succeed in retarding the debilitating progression of arthritic disease. Most, in fact, speed its progression. Non-steroidal anti-inflammatory drugs (NSAIDS), frequently used to treat symptoms such as pain and inflammation, actually retard healing. People who rely on these drugs over the long term tend to be worse off than those who take nothing.

Many rheumatologists, especially in the treatment of "the arthridities," are so focused on each individual manifestation of arthritis that they can't see the forest for the trees. Alternative medicine practitioners, on the other hand, believe and specialize in seeing the forest (the big picture) as well as the trees (the symptoms). Indeed, holistic medicine as a whole acknowledges the fact that no two people are the same, and that the different variations of arthritis are simply due to each individual's unique genomic expression of a commonality of causes.

The Inflammatory-Pain Cycle

Bracing (the unconscious total-body chronic muscle tension described in Chapter 6) is univerally present among arthritics. Bracing puts significant stress directly on the ligaments and joints, resulting in inflammation. This creates a vicious cycle because the inflammation signals for more blood, which in turn brings a greater immune response to the inflamed areas, which in turn results in even *more* muscle tension and pain. Finally, the increased blood circulation to the inflamed areas results in a chronically decreased blood supply to the gastrointestinal tract, setting the stage for leaky gut syndrome (LGS). In turn, LGS tends to create intracellular magnesium deficiencies of such magnitude that they cannot easily be resolved by diet or oral supplementation alone.

Fibromyalgia (also called fibromyositis) is a condition involving pain and soreness in the muscles and ligaments that persists over long periods of time. Fibromyalgia is one example of a relatively "new" disorder being more and more commonly diagnosed by conventional medicine. Once I became aware of the role of magnesium deficiency in arthritic disorders, I began looking for it and found that nearly *every* fibromyalgia patient that I tested had low intracellular magnesium levels. Magnesium deficiency causes muscle tension *all by itself*—whether a person has arthritis or not.

Sometimes "arthritis" is present in a single joint as opposed to being widespread. The knees are especially susceptible to problems for several reasons. First, they have to bear the entire weight of your body with every step. Also, they have long bones that place leverage on each side of the joint. Knee bones also "stick out" enough to make them more prone to injury. Long-distance running is a fad which began just a few decades ago, and has only recently proven extremely damaging to the knees. For many people, chronic knee problems are due to one or more injuries, most of which could have been prevented. For others, a combination of longstanding bracing, the wear and tear of carrying around excess weight and/or bending and moving without proper form are to blame.

Therapeutic Approaches to Healing

Besides correcting any magnesium deficiency and obesity issues, several other therapeutic approaches will be of great benefit to the arthritic. These include eliminating tobacco; performing gentle stretching, underwater exercises, and Feldenkrais Method or Alexander Technique; getting a Rolfing or massage series; and following certain dietary restrictions. The first approach, eliminating tobacco, is self-explanatory.

The next approach, performing gentle stretching, is crucial for lessening pain and improving mobility. Stretching must be done correctly to get the most benefit with the least risk of injury. If the stretches are uncomfortable, you are likely performing them incorrectly. I recommend the technique in *Synergetics,* available as both a book and a DVD by Taylor and Joanna Hay.[1] For the expenditure of only twelve minutes twice a day, I predict you will find everything else you are doing for your arthritis will work better.

The next recommendations are to engage in regular underwater exercise, which allows anyone with connective tissue inflammatory conditions to receive aerobic benefits not otherwise possible because the water eliminates much of the gravity that stresses the joints. Most communities have inexpensive public service programs providing training and facilities for underwater therapy (such as high school pools, YMCA or YWCA and year-round public pools). For added benefit, I recommend learning either Feldenkrais Method or the Alexander Technique (choose one or the other), and putting it into practice in your everyday life.[2]

In addition, Rolfing—a form of deep fascial tissue massage—has proven to be remarkably effective in returning debilitated arthritic patients to more active lives.[3] Fascial tissue or "fascia" is the connective tissues between your muscles. I believe that Rolfing should be the first course of action routinely prescribed by rheumatologists. Unfortunately, since Ida Rolf was not a licensed physician (meaning Rolfing wasn't developed by a member of the physicians' "union"), she and her method have been classed along with the rest of the competition. If Rolfing is not a viable option for you, great benefits can also be obtained with a series of three 90-minute total-body deep-tissue therapeutic massages per week for two weeks in a row.

Eliminating Dietary Culprits

Finally, there is a definite relationship between diet and arthritis that is often overlooked. Begin by eliminating nightshade foods (peppers, white potatoes, eggplant, tomatoes, cayenne and paprika). In about one third of people diagnosed with an arthritic disorder, joint aches and swelling are simply reactions to the solanine found in these nightshade foods. Since solanine exacerbates connective tissue tension, it is certainly worth conducting a trial elimination. It may take up to six months of total elimination to experience the full benefits.[4]

Due to the LGS caused by bracing, many arthritic patients find they have gastrointestinal problems, therefore most also have food hypersensitivities (known or unknown).* Immune reactions to common dietary proteins such as gluten (wheat) and casein (dairy) *directly* affect the connective tissues, therefore a trial of total elimination of all traces may well be beneficial.[5] Gastrointestinal problems are frequently blamed on arthritis medications, however most patients will recall they had some of these problems prior to beginning the medications, which simply made the gastrointestinal issues worse.

I first became aware of the potential connections between diet and arthritis after reading a research study by Marshall Mandell, MD. He was able to demonstrate a 75% improvement in the symptoms of his patients with rheumatoid arthritis within six days of starting a supervised water fast. After the sixth day (by which time the improvements were obvious), foods were reintroduced in a controlled manner, one at a time, to determine which foods were causing symptoms for any individual. With results like this, the burden of proof now shifts to those naysayers who continually deny the possibility of any such dietary relationship. No one is suggesting that diet is the *cause* of arthritis. Rather, it is the way people with LGS digest and absorb their food (LGS) that explains how diet might *influence* arthritis.[6]

---

* See Chapter 7: *Leaky Gut Syndrome* and Chapter 27: *Elimination/Provocation Diet.*

In addition to the recommendations given so far, supplementation with essential fatty acids (EFAs), certain antioxidants, glucosamine sulphate, MSM (methylsulfonylmethane) and alfalfa tablets have all been shown to be beneficial adjunctive therapies for anyone suffering from arthritic disorders.

Synergistic Supplements

The first supplement that arthritics will find almost universally helpful is essential fatty acids (EFAs), the use of which is described in Chapter 29. EFAs have been found to significantly alter the two main physiological pathways identified with arthritic inflammation. Omega 3 inhibits the prostaglandin II series that tends to cause arthritic inflammation, and omega 6 promotes the prostaglandin I series, which inhibits arthritic inflammation.[7] Most people in our country are more deficient in omega 3s than omega 6s.

Secondly, there are two major antioxidants that will not only help most arthritics, but recently have even been accepted by most conventional medical authorities as useful in preventing heart disease and cancer. Vitamin C is the major water-soluble antioxidant, and vitamin E is the major fat-soluble antioxidant. Antioxidants work by neutralizing the free radicals that are mostly responsible for the damage involved in all degenerative diseases. I recommend taking at least 800 IU of natural vitamin E (mixed tocopherols) and two grams of esterified vitamin C daily. These doses are fairly inexpensive and completely safe, and most people with arthritis will have noticeable benefits within a month of starting these two antioxidants together.

Next, veterinarians have been using glucosamine sulphate (also spelled "sulfate") in arthritic animals with remarkable success for the past few decades. Today, that recommendation is almost universal. My holistic vet began recommending glucosamine for my arthritic dog over twenty years ago, and within three months I saw no more observable symptoms. Most allopathic doctors are finally acknowledging the effectiveness of glucosamine in people (the jury is still out on chondroitin). I recommend taking 750 mg of glucosamine sulphate twice a day, the *only* supplement that has shown evidence of joint damage reversal, proven by X-ray, in conventional medical studies. No arthritis medications prescribed today can make this claim.

And finally, MSM and alfalfa tablets are two other nutritional supplements worth looking into for anyone suffering from arthritic conditions. Both can be safely added to your regimen and taken according to the directions on the label. Plan on giving all of the above about three months to achieve their full effect.

Keep in mind that all nutritional substances tend to work together synergistically. Correcting one deficiency will naturally make any other supplements you take work a little better. Given that the body requires at least forty additional trace micronutrients, I recommend taking high-quality multiple vitamin, mineral and essential amino acid supplements. Keep in mind there's no such thing as a good "one-a-day" multiple, so any supplement claiming to have it all in one tablet is not one I would take. To provide an adequate supply of all needed nutrients, a "one-a-day" would have to be the size of a ping pong ball! Do your research and choose only superior-quality supplements, especially those that include "whole food concentrates" from a manufacturer with proven ingredients and results.[8]

The "Tip of the Iceberg"

As with *all* chronic health conditions, arthritic disorders can accurately be viewed as just the "tip of the iceberg" of what is going on in the rest of your physiology due to the very same causes. This explains why so many arthritis patients also have allergies, chronic fatigue syndrome, PMS, colitis and other *seemingly* unrelated conditions.

As with all chronic health conditions, the underlying cause of arthritic disorders is rooted in the overwhelming stored stress-effect in the hypothalamus (which leads to bracing, which leads to LGS, which leads to inflammation and so forth). In the long run, the cheapest and most effective approach is to learn and practice the 3LS Wellness lifestyle outlined in detail in Section IV of this book. Since none of the options detailed in this chapter will interfere with any conventional treatment you may be receiving, you have nothing to lose but your symptoms in trying them.

CHAPTER 17

Cancer

It is impossible for anyone to begin to learn what he believes he already knows.

~ Epictetus
(Greek Stoic philosopher, 55 AD–135 AD)

The "War on Cancer"

"Cancer" is a general term used to describe more than one hundred diseases, all of which are characterized by the uncontrolled growth of abnormal cells. Some types of cancer cells grow and spread only locally (such as basal cell carcinoma of the skin), whereas other types of cancer cells metastasize and spread, via the bloodstream and lymphatic system, to other areas of the body.

Twenty years after the United States government under President Nixon announced the launch of the "War on Cancer," *Scientific American* published a major article entitled, "We are Losing the War on Cancer."[1] This came as no surprise to me. Although in recent years the allopathic medical paradigm has finally begun to acknowledge the importance of a healthy lifestyle for cancer prevention, this particular "war" has been based entirely on our system's track record for approaching dis-ease from a "treatment" standpoint only.[2]

Consider this: The current policy of calling a five-year survival a *cure* is, in my opinion, a cruel misrepresentation of the facts. The truth is, patients with most types of cancer would survive *at least* that long with no treatment at all. Our country's current pink-ribbon, "early detection" approach to breast cancer is a good example of the well-intentioned masses buying into a campaign based on a one-sided paradigm filled with false premises, including the push for "early detection."

Early Detection? Do the Math

The theory behind early detection is that the sooner a cancer is found, the sooner treatment can begin. The goal is admirable—a higher chance for a cure. What the public isn't being told is this: Even the most conservative doctors are beginning to admit that, with rare exception, *people with most types of cancer are not living any longer with treatment than without.*

There is no doubt temporary results can be obtained through surgery, chemotherapy and radiation (cut, poison and burn). After all, can anyone deny the absence of a finger if it is chopped off? For certain types of cancer, these conventional treatment approaches can be life saving, yet they do *nothing* to reverse the bodily conditions that allowed cancer to occur in the first place. Cancer treatments may induce "remission;" however except in certain instances, they cannot be considered a "cure."

The long-term cancer survival rate statistics given by the media are based more on simple arithmetic than on the actual effectiveness of any conventional treatment. Take breast cancer for example. The earlier the cancer is detected, the more years it can be treated, and so the higher the five-year "survival" statistics will *appear* to be. However, statistics have clearly shown that the natural "survival" period from the first appearance of breast cancer cells, with no conventional treatment at all, is twenty years. That means, if breast cancer is discovered in its fifth year, the average person can expect a fifteen-year survival. If not discovered until its tenth year, the average person can expect a ten-year survival, etc. Remember, *this is with no treatment at all.*

Our country's push for routine mammography is, in and of itself, a good example of the dangers inherent in blindly following an incomplete paradigm. Mammograms expose breast tissue to high amounts of radiation, in and of itself a known carcinogen. In addition, the extreme compression aspect of a mammogram is one of the suspected causes for metastasis of any cancer cells that may be present.[3]

As if the risks of radiation and metastasis combined with the sobering long-term survival statistics weren't enough, mammograms have been known to have a 70–80% false positive rate, resulting in huge numbers of unnecessary biopsies. Mammograms *also* have a high rate of false negatives, missing as many as one in four cancers that are actually present. When a mammogram *does* accurately detect a true cancer in its early stages, the result is another patient joining the army of "treated" cancer victims earlier, therefore suffering the horrific side effects of the conventional cancer treatment paradigm for more years than they would have if the cancer were discovered later. The picture being painted for the public is quite the opposite.

Prostate cancer statistics are another example. In January 1994, a cancer researcher from the University of Chicago reported that untreated prostate cancer patients seemed to live longer, healthier lives than patients whom the allopathic medical system insisted on treating aggressively with surgery, chemotherapy and radiation. The same is true of many other types of cancer. The researcher went on to say that his conclusions were not likely to be accepted by many of his colleagues because "physicians like to feel like they are doing *something*."[4]

The Solution Is Within the Cause

Many studies conducted over the past twenty years have retrospectively shown that individuals who engage in certain behaviors have a much higher statistical incidence of various cancers. Tobacco is a well-known example. We no longer have any doubt that smoking (including passive smoke) increases the risk of respiratory cancers (lung, etc.), and that chewing tobacco increases the risk of mouth and pharyngeal cancers. We've also discovered that engaging in intercourse at an early age increases the risk of cervical cancer, drinking alcohol increases the risk of pancreatic cancer, and eating red meat increases the risk of colorectal cancer.[5]

Not only are most cancers *preventable*, but the same expedients that prevent cancer are also very helpful adjuncts once cancer is present. Cancer, like most chronic dis-ease, is much more likely to occur in people with poor immunity. If I were to be diagnosed with cancer, I would learn everything possible about how my current lifestyle might be contributing to my susceptibility, and do something about that, *first*. I would pay close attention to achieving and maintaining a healthy pH balance in my body and then, I would give my immune system the very best support by practicing the 3LS Wellness lifestyle described in Section IV of this book. And finally, I would live my life, joyfully, one day at a time.

When it comes to cancer prevention, one supplement worth mentioning is selenium. In 1997, it was reported that the four most common cancers in this country would each be reduced by over 50% if people would just supplement their diets with 200 micrograms of selenium per day.[6] This is not a case of "if some is good, more is better." Too much selenium is toxic. Given that careful supplementation of selenium is simple, inexpensive and without negative side effects, why isn't this common knowledge? Perhaps part of the reason is because the American Cancer Society, the world's wealthiest *non-profit* institution, "is fixated on damage control—diagnosis and treatment—and basic molecular biology, with indifference and even hostility to cancer prevention."[7]

The Cancer Prevention Coalition, on the other hand, is a nationwide alliance of leading independent experts in cancer prevention. Its goal is to "reduce escalating cancer rates through a comprehensive strategy of outreach, public education, advocacy and public policy initiatives to establish prevention as the nation's foremost cancer policy."[8] The Cancer Prevention Coalition is wisely pushing for more money to be funneled into prevention research rather than the billions currently being funneled into conventional detection and treatment approaches.

Positive Biopsy: Treatment Risks and Benefits

Cancer is definitively diagnosed by obtaining a sample (biopsy) of the suspected area and examining the cells at a lab. *Negative* biopsy reports can sometimes be wrong. However, unless a specimen is somehow mixed up with that of another patient, a *positive* biopsy for any cancer is considered 100% accurate. In other words, cancer can be missed (especially depending on the method by which the sample was obtained), but cancer cells cannot be invented under the microscope. If they are seen, they are there.

If you have been diagnosed with cancer of any kind, any treatment *must* be judged on the basis of long-term results, including weighing *risks* versus *benefits*. Different cancers respond to different approaches. Some examples of the types of cancer that respond best to conventional treatments include testicular cancer, Hodgkin's lymphoma and acute lymphatic leukemia. For other cancers, the best approach or combination of approaches is highly individual. Much depends on the *type, stage* and *aggressiveness* of the cancer cells found. For low to average aggressiveness, I personally, would do nothing conventional.

If you or a loved one has been diagnosed with cancer, I strongly recommend getting in touch with the Cancer Control Society along with one of the inpatient Cancer Treatment Centers of America.[9] Both are at the forefront in combining conventional cancer treatment with complementary approaches, and both can assist you and your doctor in sorting through what's best for your individual circumstances. You are treated as an active participant in deciding which course(s) of action to take—the only way it *should* be.

I know of few conventional physicians with the courage to openly investigate the type of information given in this chapter. Indeed, given that the proven statistics are so opposite to what is taught in medical school and what is being promoted in the media, only the most forward-thinking patients who do their own research will ever have an opportunity to become aware of these facts.

The same goes for the general public, many of whom are not ready to face the facts. Those who simply follow what "the doctor" says will never be aware of the available alternatives. The fact that you are reading this book demonstrates that you are among the most open-minded and proactive individuals. If you should ever happen to be diagnosed with cancer, you will have far greater odds of not only surviving, but of enjoying a much higher quality of life than those who have never been exposed to the facts presented in this chapter.

CHAPTER 18

Acne and Sebaceous Cysts

The truth that makes men free is for the most part the truth which men prefer not to hear.

~ Herbert Agar
(Pulitzer Prize-winning journalist, 1897–1980)

Acne: The Hormone Connection

Acne is an *extremely* common condition of adolescence, the period of life when the most dramatic changes in endocrinological (hormonal) function take place. Among these changes is the formation of sebaceous glands under the arms, on the face, on the upper chest and back, and in the groin area. Have you ever noticed that young children rarely have body odor, even when they haven't bathed for several days? That's because sebaceous glands are not even *present* prior to the onset of puberty. They are the source of body odor as well as those infamous sex pheromones.

Sebaceous glands make oily secretions (sebum) that serve to lubricate your skin, keeping it moist and flexible. When hormones are out of balance, however, the sebum can become thicker than normal, clogging pores and leading to blackheads, whiteheads, pimples ("zits") and cysts. Since hormones are naturally out of whack during puberty, acne is pretty much to be expected. Acne that continues into *adulthood*, however, is another story. If you are an adult who is still struggling with chronic acne, have you ever stopped to wonder *why* it has persisted?

The common thread in both adolescent *and* adult acne is hormonal imbalance. This undeniable connection is especially easy to observe in women. For example, "breakouts" are more common during the premenstrual phase of a woman's monthly cycle. During pregnancy, some women will develop acne for the first time in their lives, whereas others will be pleasantly surprised to find their former acne problem clearing up. Birth control pills have been known to affect acne, exacerbating the condition in some women and improving it in others. Even the most genetically-affected women who have battled acne their entire adult lives often find it completely disappears at menopause. Of course, *anyone* who is genetically predisposed—both male and female—has the potential to manifest chronic adult acne.

Like Parent, Like Child

It's easy to observe that acne tends to "run in the family." However, any genetic predisposition should be thought of only as a *tendency*—not an absolute. Anyone battling acne as an adult has to have a reason (a cause *aside* from genetics) for why the glandular imbalance has persisted beyond puberty. The genetic aspect simply determines why one person will develop acne whereas someone else, with different genetics, will develop thyroid disease, ovarian cysts or depression instead—from the very same causes. *None* of these conditions are inevitable!

Regardless of the outward manifestation, whether it be acne or any other dis-ease, the common denominator is the same—accumulation of overwhelming stress-effect storage in the hypothalamus. In the case of genetically predisposed adults with chronic acne, this hypothalamic burden causes the hormonal imbalance, which *then* causes the acne condition. In adolescents with significant acne, the hypothalamic burden simply adds to an *already* imbalanced hormonal system.

Of course, since chronic acne manifests outwardly on the face and body, it can have potentially devastating effects on one's personal appearance and self-esteem. The result—an understandably desperate search for *anything* that will "clear up" the skin. As is the case with *all* chronic health conditions, any "treatment" approach that fails to simultaneously take the root cause of the problem into account will naturally fail to permanently solve it, each and every time.

I have yet to see chronic acne permanently *cured* by any of the acne treatment products (such as medications, creams and cleansers) offered by dermatologists, drug stores and infomercials. This includes oral antibiotics, steroid injections, isotretinoin, all topical antimicrobials, retinoids, astringents, benzoyl peroxide and salicylic acid. During adolescence, acne treatments can only help to manage symptoms until the person grows out of it. As we have seen, some people *never* grow out of it.

The Irony of Acne Antibiotics

As a newly practicing physician, before I understood that treating the *symptoms* of acne rarely provided more than temporary benefits (and also risked potentially serious side effects), I routinely prescribed the antibiotic tetracycline for my acne patients. Today, I never recommend antibiotic treatment for acne *unless* there is a severe flare-up that has become secondarily infected. Even then, antibiotics can often be avoided by using hot compresses for a day or two before calling the doctor.* If antibiotics truly *are* indicated, they should only be used until the secondary infection is eliminated (a few days at most, as long as the hot compresses are continued).

When long-term doses of antibiotics are prescribed (one month or more), your doctor is attempting to treat one of the acne *mechanisms*, not the secondarily infected acne. For the acne mechanism, it takes at least one month for results to begin to show and 3–6 months to receive the full benefits. It may even seem as though your problem has been solved. After about a year, though, the average person will be disappointed to learn firsthand that antibiotics aren't going to work forever. Acne nearly always returns, and the patient goes back to square one—searching for the *next* "miracle cure."

Once I learned enough to begin looking at the big picture of acne from a holistic point of view, I began to see how taking long-term antibiotics creates a truly ironic situation. People with acne nearly always have leaky gut syndrome (LGS). Antibiotics destroy the "friendly flora" (good bacteria) in the gastrointestinal tract, making one highly susceptible to dysbiosis. Dysbiosis, in turn, contributes to Candida-related syndrome (C-RS). In other words, long-term antibiotics have created *additional* stressful factors,

* See Chapter 30: *Avoiding Unnecessary Antibiotics* and Chapter 31: *Hot Compresses.*

besides your genetics, that are now perpetuating the vicious cycle. The acne condition often becomes even *worse* than it was before the antibiotic treatment began, leading some people to take even more desperate measures.

Isotretinoin (Accutane)

Isotretinoin (generally sold under the brand name "Accutane") is a systemic drug with the potential for severe and devastating side effects. It can stunt a teenager's growth and cause drastic birth defects in an unborn child. It has also been linked to baldness, fatigue, joint pains, liver damage, depression and suicide. I know of few people who would take isotretinoin after having read all the facts about it in the package insert or Physician's Desk Reference (PDR).

Dermatologists have been trained to reserve isotretinoin *only* for patients with severe cystic acne, *only* as a last resort, and *only* after several precautions have been meticulously taken. Not all dermatologists heed these guidelines. Anyone who chooses to take this drug must be given a clear understanding of the serious risks and must be clearly told that even *this* is a treatment, not a cure, for acne.

In my opinion, by far the worst side effect of isotretinoin (or *any* conventional treatment approach to acne) is not even mentioned in any of the warning literature. That is, if it works without serious consequences to your overall health, you no longer have any incentive to take your acne as a message. It would be foolish to think your problem has been solved just because your skin is clear. If your bodymind's message of sending you acne is not heard, it will eventually shout louder. The next message may be one you cannot ignore. Acne sufferers who mistakenly believe only their skin is affected will pay the price of reduced health throughout their lives.

The following are several safe, effective holistic treatments you can use while simultaneously doing what it takes to reverse the underlying cause of your acne. With this comprehensive approach, you can enjoy significant short-term relief of acne symptoms *as well as* an overall elevation in health. Keep in mind that none of the holistic treatments given in this chapter truly constitute a *cure* for acne, but they can go a long way toward providing relief while you are simultaneously doing what it takes (the 3LS of Wellness) to achieve that cure.

EFAs and Oily Skin

Acne is at least partially related to errors in fat metabolism, which explains why many people notice their skin becomes oilier after eating greasy or high-fat foods. The connection between greasy foods and greasy skin often leads people to conclude they should avoid all dietary fats and oils, which couldn't be further from the truth. Instead, the right *kinds* of oils are necessary for normal metabolism of all fats, and people with chronic acne have a genetic need for more essential fatty acids (EFAs) than the general population. When you are deficient in EFAs, any increase in dietary fat intake results in your body trying to excrete fat in one of the few ways it can—through the sebaceous glands.

Chapter 29 gives detailed information and instructions on how to determine your ideal therapeutic and maintenance doses, however it's important to describe here how EFAs play a role in acne specifically. EFA deficiencies cause the oily secretions from sebaceous glands (sebum) to become thicker and stickier than normal. As these thickened secretions try to flow to the surface of the skin through the tiny ducts, they start to dry and oxidize from exposure to the air, causing the formation of a hard plug. A plugged duct, however, does not stop the gland from continuing to do what it is programmed to do—make more sebum.

EFA supplementation helps the secretions return to normal fluidity (thickness) so they are less quickly oxidized or dried into plugs. Also, with EFA supplementation, the first thing you will notice is a drastic reduction in the oiliness of your complexion because fat metabolism will normalize. Given that so many important metabolic functions inside the body (aside from the skin) are dependent upon a healthy level of EFAs, you'll likely notice improvement in your overall health as well.

Vitamin B5 and Zinc

Pantothenic acid (vitamin B5) is another alternative treatment receiving increasing attention among acne sufferers. Research published in *The Journal of Orthomolecular Medicine* has expanded our understanding about the specific role hormones play in acne causation, showing that chronic acne sufferers are often deficient in coenzyme A, an important enzyme involved in the synthesis of sex hormones and fatty acid metabolism.[1] Of the three components that make up coenzyme A, vitamin B5 is the only component that must be obtained from the diet. Deficiency forces the body to use any available B5 for the most important functions (sex hormone synthesis), thereby neglecting the least important functions (fatty acid metabolism).

In a recent study, remarkable results were seen when daily megadoses of ten grams of B5 were given to chronic acne sufferers.[2] Several of my online bulletin board participants experimented with taking 5–10 grams per day and indeed reported an amazing reduction in the amount and severity of their acne. Although such a large dose of B5 appears to be safe, mega-dosing on any one B vitamin has the potential to induce a relative deficiency in all the other B vitamins. Therefore, I recommend including a good balanced B complex alongside your B5 supplement regimen.

Zinc is another supplement I have found almost universally helpful for acne sufferers. Zinc is best taken with vitamins C, E and A, in addition to the EFA protocol already described. I recommend beginning with therapeutic doses higher than what will be needed for maintenance once benefits are realized. Start with 30 mg of zinc twice a day, 2000 mg esterified vitamin C twice a day, 1000 IU of natural vitamin E (mixed tocopherols) once a day, and 50,000 IU of natural vitamin A once a day.

The skin replaces itself every four weeks. Therefore, take all recommended supplements at these doses for at least eight weeks to ensure stable benefits. At that point, you can experiment with cutting them down little by little every eight weeks until you begin to see acne symptoms returning. At that point, simply go back up to your most recent lowest effective doses for maintenance.

Next, just as some people have a genetic predisposition toward chronic acne, others are genetically predisposed to its close cousin—chronic and recurrent sebaceous cysts.

Sebaceous Cysts

Sebaceous cysts are caused when an already blocked gland continues to accumulate sebum, causing pressure to build up.* Soon, the lining of the

* Sebaceous cysts that form in the armpits are almost always caused by the use of antiperspirants. For these, see "Antiperspirants: Why I *Never* Use Them" in Chapter 22: *Excessive Body Odor.*

gland gets pushed into the duct, causing infection, damage and permanent blockage. Their formation can often be mechanically prevented with daily gentle exfoliation of the skin which will help remove early developing plugs. If any new cysts *do* begin to form (signaled by pain, swelling and redness), apply moist, hot compresses at the very first sign to have the best chance of preventing it from reaching the stage of permanence.

Once a sebaceous cyst reaches the size of a pea, the mechanics of pressure can prevent its resolution, and the damaged gland may require surgical removal. Sebaceous cysts should never be surgically removed while infected. At the very first sign of infection, begin the hot compresses as directed. Lancing and draining an infected cyst is also not recommended because it almost *guarantees* its return.

A physician who is knowledgeable about the causation and structure of sebaceous cysts can typically remove one under local anesthetic in less than fifteen minutes. This type of surgery must be done very carefully if it is to be permanently successful. A small knick is made in the skin, then tiny forceps are used to carefully peel out the sack (similar to removing a pea from its skin). Done correctly, most incisions won't even need a stitch unless they are on the face, in which case you may want to consider having the procedure performed by a plastic surgeon.

Be sure to find a knowledgeable and *skillful* physician who has experience with performing this surgical procedure. If the cyst ruptures during removal, a large piece of surrounding tissue will then *also* likely need to be removed because any scraps of the lining left behind will just continue making sebum, causing another cyst to form. Failure to do the procedure properly causes a scarred wall, making any future surgical attempt much more difficult.

The very same holistic approaches outlined in this chapter for preventing and treating acne will also work for sebaceous cysts. After about three months of following the EFA protocol alone, you will notice a great reduction in the formation of new cysts. After about a year, there should be no new cysts forming at all.

Beauty from the Inside Out

This book is about going beyond the mindset of simply treating the outward symptoms of dis-ease. I continually encourage people to deal with *why* they still have acne and sebaceous cysts rather than desperately seeking something (*anything!*) to clear up their skin. As with all the other chronic health conditions discussed in this book, the cure for these problems (including oily skin) can only be achieved by taking the pressure off the hypothalamic FOF storage.

In all my years of experience, I have yet to see any person with these types of persistent skin problems, regardless of age, that did not clear up completely within 6–12 months of practicing the 3LS Wellness guidelines outlined in Section IV of this book. When you address your acne and sebaceous cysts with a Wellness approach, what you are really doing is reversing your underlying dysautonomia and endocrinopathy, both of which are much more serious conditions in the long run.

CHAPTER 19

Fungal Infections of the Feet

One of the first duties of the physician
is to educate the masses not to take medicine.

~ Sir William Osler
(Canadian physician, historian and author, 1849–1919)

There's a Fungus Among Us!

The little rhyme is true. Fungi are literally lurking everywhere, all around us, all the time. Despite their prevalence, the only way fungi can live and grow is by feeding on dead organic material—their ecological niche in our world. It just so happens the surface of your skin is dead, as is all your visible nail tissue. Considering that fungi thrive especially well in warm, dark and moist environments, it is no surprise that the feet, mouth and vagina ("yeast infections") are among their favorite places of residence.

This chapter will focus on athlete's foot and fungal toenails, the two most common types of fungal foot infections for which millions of people seek treatment each year. The solutions given here require no medical supervision, are completely safe and effective, and practically free. For these same reasons, they are neither taught nor promoted by the conventional medical paradigm, nor featured on television infomercials. In fact, these home remedies would wipe out millions of dollars in physician consultation fees and prescription pharmaceutical treatments.

I will begin by describing the three most significant factors that prevent fungi from establishing themselves on your feet: hygiene, moisture and immunity. Until or unless these preventive factors are understood and attended to, any cure for fungal foot infections is likely to be temporary at best.

Prevention: Three Critical Factors

The first factor in preventing fungal foot infections involves the amount of dead organic material available on your feet. My mother used to say, "Be sure to wash and dry between your toes!" Mom was right (of course). If you aren't carefully washing, drying and buffing your feet and toes with every bath or shower, using a fresh clean terrycloth wash cloth and towel each time, your feet will be a feeding ground for fungus. Terrycloth was originally *designed* for buffing off dead skin cell layers, so the best towels and washcloths for this purpose are usually the least expensive ones with the most texture.

The second factor has to do with how much moisture is continuously on your feet. Keep in mind that the sweatier your feet are, the more moisture you will accumulate inside your socks and shoes. Although it's normal for humans to sweat to some degree, the more stress-effect storage you have, the sweatier you will be. Even if excessive sweating isn't an issue, modern shoes create that perfect warm, dark, moist environment that fungi love so much. The more your feet are exposed to the air, the better—so the obvious solution is to go barefoot as much as possible (even during your lunch hour at work). When you *must* wear socks and shoes, change your socks as often as needed to keep your feet dry throughout the day.

Finally, the third factor involves the strength of your immune system, which is in charge of defending your body against invaders. The hypothalamic fight-or-flight (FOF) stress-effect load described in Chapters 5 and 6 directly affects immune strength, *as well as* circulation and sweat volume. Infections of any kind are due to a combination of your resistance (immunity) *and* the concentration of the invading organisms. The FOF response that reduces circulation to your extremities (making them chronically cold) also decreases the immune reserves available to kill any fungal spores that might be lurking on your feet.

Athlete's Foot (Tinea Pedis)

A simple rule we doctors learn in medical school is that rashes on the tops of the feet are nearly always caused by allergy, and rashes on the bottoms of the feet or between the toes are nearly always caused by fungus. Athlete's foot is so named because it most commonly affects athletes—those who spend the most time with their feet confined in warm, dark, sweaty socks and shoes.

Athlete's foot infections most commonly begin between the toes (preventable by daily buffing) then make their way along the bottoms and sides of the feet. Once firmly established, the fungi become vigorous enough to begin growing into the deeper layers of the skin, causing painful, itchy breaks.

By strictly following the preventive foot hygiene rules already outlined, you will be *very* unlikely to get athlete's foot in the first place. Once the infection is present, however, preventive techniques alone are rarely enough to reverse it. Discard and replace your heavily contaminated shoes, then begin following the hygiene protocol. With that alone, nearly any topical anti-fungal medication will easily resolve the problem because the factors that caused it are no longer present. Unfortunately, this is the vital piece of information almost never given to patients seeing their doctors for athlete's foot.

It's not as important *which* topical anti-fungal substance is used so much as *how* it is used. The least expensive 2% miconazole nitrate powders and creams are usually sufficient. Desenex is one example of such a product. To guarantee the highest rate of cure, follow this protocol faithfully: You will need two pairs of clean dry socks each day. In the evening, wash and dry your feet *thoroughly*, buffing between the toes. Once completely dry (expose them to the air as long as possible), apply Desenex cream liberally to the affected areas and all adjacent skin. Next, liberally sprinkle Desenex powder inside a clean, dry pair of socks. Wear the socks all night and repeat the entire procedure in the morning.

Skin replaces itself about every four weeks. In the case of athlete's foot, I recommend continuing treatment for at least one week *after* your skin appears completely normal (about five weeks total). If treatment is discontinued too soon, athlete's foot is much more likely to recur. Of course, if you are not following the prevention protocol both during treatment and thereafter, it will probably recur no matter what you do.

Fungal Toenails (Onychomycosis)

Onychomycosis is another common fungal condition that typically presents as an unsightly thickening and discoloration of the toenails. Nearly all fungal nail infections begin at the tips of the nails (the portion that you trim off) and work their way down to the growing base. The debris that collects under the toenail is a near perfect culture medium for fungi, so you can imagine why the big toenail is the most common one affected. When toenail debris is not cleaned out with a nail file at least once a week (daily is better), it is little wonder the nail finally becomes infected.

Once established, fungal toenails tend to be permanent unless properly addressed. Since several other nail conditions (such as psoriatic nails), look similar to the unaided eye, you may want to ask your physician to send a nail sample to the lab for culture and microscopic examination before embarking on the minimum six-month fungal treatment course.

Conventional medicine offers two basic options for this vexing problem: surgical removal of the toenail, and/or many months of expensive (and often dangerous) oral antifungal medications. Surgery is not only painful, it also cannot reach the growing portion of the nail lying deep beneath the skin. Side effects of the most commonly prescribed oral antifungal drugs include headache, diarrhea, liver failure and death.[1] That's a *huge* price to pay in your quest for a healthy toenail. And, what the drug companies don't tell you is this: Unless the infection has progressed to the point that the fungi has spread to the live tissues, oral antifungals can't actually *get* to the fungi because dead tissue (and therefore the fungi that live and grow on it) is not accessible via the bloodstream.

This seemingly impossible condition really does have a safe, effective and inexpensive solution, which is practically free and almost never fails to work—vinegar.[2] Simply go to any grocery store and purchase the cheapest 4–5% acetic acid distilled vinegar you can find. The more expensive, higher acidity vinegars are no more effective and can cause irritation in sensitive people. Then, obtain a small glass dropper bottle and follow the instructions below.

Vinegar: 2 Drops, Twice a Day

Before you begin, it is helpful to gain a thorough understanding of what, exactly, you are working to accomplish. There is no such thing as a "quick fix" for toenail fungus, and that goes for both conventional *and* holistic treatments. Vinegar treatment is based on the fact that fungi do not like an acid environment. All *any* fungal treatment can do, whether applied topically or taken orally, is inhibit the growth of fungi in the live tissue formed on that particular day. When it comes to fungal toenails, the goal is to keep the living, forming nail tissue (the tissue you cannot see) *acidic*. This is easily accomplished by applying two drops of vinegar at the growing base of the nail (cuticle)—twice a day without fail.

The key to success is to follow the protocol exactly. Don't use more than two drops and don't soak your toes in the vinegar, either. Soaking the toes adds too much moisture, which being the friend of the fungus, is counterproductive. Since all *visible* nail tissue is dead, there is also no need to pour, drop, wipe or swab vinegar on the toenail itself. Immediately after application, the vinegar microscopically invades the base of the nail's growing matrix, so you don't have to wait for the vinegar to absorb or dry before going about your business.

Vinegar Treatment, or . . . "How to Make Your Feet Smell Like a Tossed Salad"

Simply fill a dropper bottle with the *cheapest* distilled vinegar that can be found at any grocery store. The vinegar that works is 95–96% water. Apply 2 drops at the growing base of the nail twice a day, without fail, every morning and every night.

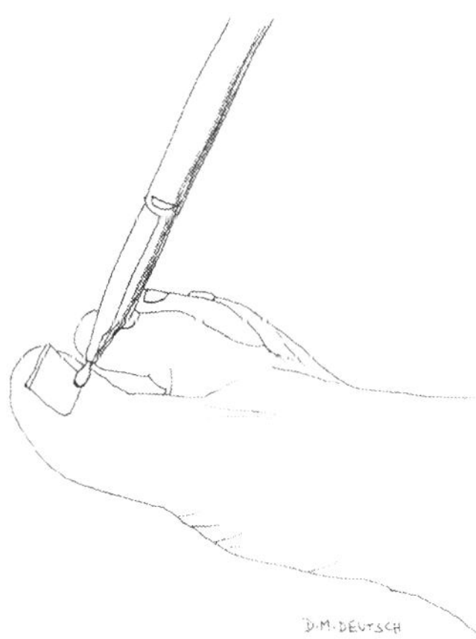

Drops should be placed on the area where the toenail base emerges from under the cuticle.

Do whatever it takes to ensure you don't forget your twice-a-day vinegar treatment. Set alarms or post reminders for yourself if needed. If even *one* application is missed, the nail tissue that grew on *that day* may not be resistant. The fungi could then potentially jump from the infected portion of the nail to the new healthy (but not resistant) nail. I cannot stress this point enough—do not miss a single application! As the new nail is slowly being formed, day after day, you must continuously create that acidic environment until the infected nail literally grows itself right off the body.

Growing a New Healthy Nail

It is astounding how far the nail goes back under the skin (all the way to the bone). This hidden portion of the nail doesn't even *begin* to grow normally until you start the vinegar treatment. Then, it can take anywhere from 3–6 months for the new healthy nail to start emerging from the base where you can see it for the first time! As you continue the vinegar treatment twice a day without fail, you will see more and more beautiful healthy nail emerging. As the nail grows, you will be trimming off bits of the old infected toenail until eventually, it is gone.

It takes the average person 6–12 months to grow a completely new nail. The rate of nail growth differs from person to person and there's nothing I know of that can speed it up. I have seen a few nails grow out in as little as four months and a very few that took as long as two years. Once you have a completely normal looking toenail, you *must* continue the vinegar treatment for at least one additional month (an average total of 7–13 months). If stopped too soon, the infection is likely to recur. In addition, become diligent about cleaning out the debris that collects under the nails on a regular basis for the rest of your life.

A note to nail polish fans: Polish tends to shade the nail (block out light) as well as hold moisture in. For these reasons, polish tends to be a friend of the fungus and an enemy to your nails. While it *is* possible to successfully complete vinegar treatment while wearing nail polish, I have seen many cases that would not clear until after it was discontinued. Once the nail has been normal for about a year, wearing occasional polish should be fine as long as you have deleted the other risk factors described in this chapter.

Conventional treatment options do nothing to address the underlying factors that enabled you to get a fungal infection in the first place; therefore they are also highly unlikely to effect a permanent cure. Why risk the side effects of surgery or prescription oral antifungal medications, when inexpensive, natural and completely safe alternatives are readily available? With the information in this chapter, you can *cure* your fungal foot infections as well as prevent new infections from occurring in the future.

CHAPTER 20

Acid Reflux (GERD)

It is supposed to be a secret, but I'll tell you anyway.
We doctors do nothing.
We only help and encourage the doctor within.

~ Albert Schweitzer, MD
(Nobel Peace Prize recipient, 1875–1965)

What Is "Heartburn," Anyway?

For many people, heartburn is a daily nuisance. This exceedingly common problem causes gastric contents to escape upward into the esophagus, resulting in discomfort of the upper abdominal, lower chest area. Heartburn is not a "condition" in and of itself, but rather a *symptom* of several possible conditions—the most common being hiatal hernia, acid reflux and gastroesophageal reflux disorder (GERD). Since these are all functionally the same, I will refer to them as "GERD" from here on out.

Conventional medical treatment options for GERD include surgery, special antacids to coat the esophagus and reduce stomach acidity, prescription anti-spasmodics and even tranquilizers. Except for rare cases in which surgery is performed to correct an anatomically abnormal gastroesophageal valve (typically due to trauma or severe obesity), conventional treatments tend to be dangerous, expensive and relatively ineffective. Safer and more effective measures include avoiding eating anything four hours before going to bed, abstaining from alcohol, losing any excess weight and propping the head of your bed up about eight inches. Symptoms worsen when lying down because gravity helps keep stomach acid from moving upward into the esophagus.

If you continue to suffer despite "trying everything," what follows is a simple, safe, effective and inexpensive remedy that has been the standard of treatment in traditional Chinese medicine (TCM) for thousands of years—ginger root juice.[1] With only a trip to the grocery store, a good juicer and the instructions given in this chapter, you can enjoy astonishing relief. If you don't own a juicer, see if you can borrow one from a friend. If you are skeptical, try it anyway! You have nothing to lose but your symptoms.

Ginger Root Juice Remedy

At the fruit and vegetable section of your local grocery store, select two pounds of fresh ginger root. The heavier the root, the more juice there is in it. Bring your purchase home and run it through a juicer (not a blender), and then store all the juice in a jar in your refrigerator. Freshly juiced ginger root will stay potent for at least six weeks if kept refrigerated in a tightly-sealed jar. You will notice some settling in the bottom, which you can safely ignore.

Every morning, immediately upon arising (on an empty stomach and at least one hour before eating), take one teaspoon of the juice straight. At first, it may feel like you have just swallowed 200-proof alcohol, but the warming sensation will last only a few seconds and cause you no harm. Continue this for three weeks in a row. Within a few short days you will already be noticing some relief. Ginger root juice is not a painkiller, so any improvement in symptoms is a measure of the actual healing process.

If you truly find the straight juice intolerable, you can experiment with diluting it half and half with water, but expect less dramatic results. A small percentage of people will experience relief simply drinking ginger ale or ginger tea, however I like to recommend what works for the largest percentage of people, and that is the straight ginger root juice.

I first learned about this remedy from the Chinese medicine specialist who was a member of the team of practitioners at my Holistic Medical Centre. Once I began recommending the remedy to my own patients, *all* of them reported back to me that they had been "cured." In truth, ginger root juice cannot technically be called a cure because it does nothing about preventing future episodes. With or without treatment, non-structural GERD is a condition of remissions and exacerbations. If you have another exacerbation in the future, begin the ginger root juice treatment immediately. By starting as soon as symptoms return, you will only need to take it for a few days. If you wait until your symptoms have been around for months, you will likely need the full three weeks of therapy all over again.

It is not necessary to discontinue any conventional therapy while trying the ginger root juice remedy, and I do not recommend you do so. Just be sure to avoid taking antacids within one hour before, and two hours after, swallowing the ginger root juice. Once you notice your symptoms are gone, you can *then* discuss stopping your medications with the doctor who prescribed them.

If your doctor has recommended surgery for your GERD, try this remedy first. Chances are after three weeks of taking the ginger root juice as directed, neither you nor your surgeon will be interested in going through with the procedure. If you do *not* experience complete remission of symptoms after using the remedy exactly as described, then you have either been misdiagnosed or you have more going on than GERD alone. Left unchecked, GERD can progress into a more serious condition called Barrett's esophagus. This precancerous condition, which forms little nests of acid-producing cells above the gastroesophageal valve, only occurs in individuals who first had simple GERD.

As with all chronic conditions, think of GERD as a message your bodymind is trying to send you. If nothing is done about *why* the condition occurred in the first place, your bodymind will eventually shout louder by sending you a more serious message (a new chronic health condition).

An *Alternative* Treatment Is Still a Treatment

Nobody can claim that GERD is a ginger root juice deficiency. Therefore, the underlying causes or the *why* of this condition must also be dealt with if the problem is to be ever truly resolved. Except in very rare instances, such as anatomical defects due to trauma, all GERD is but one aspect of leaky gut syndrome (LGS). When the gut becomes starved for blood, the variety of conditions that result simply depend upon the genetic and constitutional makeup of the patient.

If you get nothing else out of this chapter, my hope is you at least begin to stop looking at GERD (or any chronic condition) as an isolated condition. Think of the ginger root juice remedy as an inexpensive, safe and effective way to become asymptomatic *while* you are dealing with the underlying causes of your condition. By following the 3LS Wellness protocol outlined in Section IV of this book, your rewards will reach far beyond a permanent cure for GERD.

CHAPTER 21

Constipation and Stool Withholding

In the middle of difficulty lies opportunity.

~ Albert Einstein
(Father of modern physics, 1879–1955)

Constipation: A Matter of Lifestyle

Constipation can be defined as stools that are infrequent (less than once a day), hardened and/or difficult to pass. The average refined American diet along with our ever-increasing sedentary way of life has made constipation *so* commonplace that many people have come to view it as a "normal" aspect of life. Of course, *normal* does not necessarily mean *healthy*, and constipation is one of many potential unhealthy consequences of the lack of a Wellness lifestyle.

This chapter will focus on one of the more serious consequences of constipation: stool withholding in children. However, adults suffering from chronic constipation can achieve similar benefits by following the very same guidelines and protocol.

Can't Go? Or Maybe *Won't*

Stool withholding is a terrible problem, as anyone who has raised a child with this can attest. The cycle typically begins with a preschool-aged child having a single painful incidence of passing a very large constipated stool. The first time this happens, the unsuspecting child's eyes will get real big from the pain and surprise. If the initial experience was painful and/or frightening enough, some children will decide they aren't ever going to let *that* happen again. What began as a single episode turns into a conscious determined effort to hold all bowel movements in as long as possible. Adults know this approach would never work, but children do not.

A research study involving 482 urine-trained children between 18–30 months of age, conducted by the American Academy of Pediatrics (AAP), found that 106 of them refused to have a bowel movement in the toilet, and 29 of them developed stool withholding patterns serious enough to need the help of a pediatrician.[1] This problem cannot possibly be resolved without addressing the factors behind the initial constipation.

Even without the scenario of an original traumatizing experience with passing stool, withholding tends to be a common problem in preschoolers for complex psychological reasons not fully understood. These may include resistance or anxiety associated with toilet training, or a fear of flushing part of themselves down the toilet. Sometimes it's simply a control issue, especially if parents show anxiety over bowel training. No matter *how* the problem originally began, it can be very damaging to the child if it is left to go on for very long.

Fissures and Impaction

Once a child has been successful at withholding stool for several days in a row, there is a risk the stool could become so large that passing it causes a fissure (a painful, semi-permanent split in the skin of the anus). When a fissure is present, it is vital to prevent even *one* more large stool before the fissure has had a chance to heal completely. As with any split in the skin, if you routinely pulled the edges of the cut apart once a day, healing cannot occur.

Another risk of stool withholding is fecal impaction—a condition of having so much built-up stool that it becomes impossible to pass. Fecal impaction usually requires an emergency trip to the doctor for an experience that, I can assure you, none of you will soon forget.

Of course, the pain and fear from fissures and impaction both serve to greatly multiply the original problem. The child's logic leads him or her to an *increased* determination to avoid further trauma by continuing to withhold. Once this cycle becomes firmly established, it can go on for years if not properly addressed. Before I learned how to solve the functional causes of stool withholding, I've seen patients still suffering from this vicious cycle at the age of ten.

The good news is, this chapter offers a protocol that cannot fail to work. The very first thing that must be accomplished is ending the cycle of pain. After that point, time and your diligent efforts will eventually take care of the rest.

Ending the Cycle

As stated at the beginning of the chapter, the root cause of constipation and stool withholding has a lot to do with lifestyle choices. However, once stool withholding has reached the serious stages just described, there is too much physical and psychological trauma for diet and physical activity alone to sufficiently end the cycle. The only approach I have found to be both safe and universally effective takes considerable attention, understanding, patience and perseverance on your part. Your first goal is to establish for your child a stool soft enough, and lubricated enough, to be easy to pass, even after being withheld for 5–7 days.

The magic combination necessary to accomplish this goal is mineral oil (for softening and lubrication) and fiber (for bulk and softening). *Neither one alone will likely be sufficient once stool withholding has progressed far enough,* therefore you must use both in combination for best results.[2] Since mineral oil and fiber are not true laxatives, there's no need to worry about dependency.* Keep in mind there is tremendous variation in dosage thresholds from one individual to the next, so the proper dosages for your child can only be determined through some initial trial and error.

Part 1: Mineral Oil

The first substance is mineral oil, which unfortunately, few children will willingly take "as is." You can prepare a more palatable version by mixing

* Other than for occasional short-term use, habit-forming laxatives and suppositories are inappropriate solutions for constipation. The definition of a "laxative" is any substance that produces a bowel movement by irritation or stimulation of the colon. With repeated laxative use, the colon becomes accustomed to the "kick," and may eventually refuse to function without it—a state known as laxative dependence.

one tablespoon of mineral oil with just enough ice-cold orange juice to disguise it. (The colder the better, so keep your mineral oil in the freezer and use cold, refrigerated juice). To help the mixture blend better, you can add ¼ teaspoon baking soda and whip it all together. Serve immediately after blending and instruct the child to drink it down quickly.

Another acceptable option is emulsified flavored mineral oil, available over-the-counter from the pharmacist. However, since it is 50% water, you will need to use twice as much. If you live outside of the United States and cannot find mineral oil, look for it under the name of "liquid paraffin" or "paraffin oil."

Begin with one tablespoon of mineral oil at bedtime (or two tablespoons of emulsified flavored mineral oil), and continue increasing the dose every night as you see fit. The ultimate goal is at least two stools a day that are easy and painless to pass. It may take several days for initial results because the child will still be trying very hard to withhold. The mineral oil must be given every evening *without fail*, since it works not by absorption but by mechanically mixing with the stool that is formed that day. The correct dose for any person is just slightly less than the amount needed to produce oil floating around on the surface of the water after a bowel movement. Once you see that, simply cut back the dose about 10% for maintenance.

Offer the mineral oil at least two hours after the last meal of the day, and right before going to bed. This timing is important because mineral oil tends to carry the fat-soluble vitamins (vitamins A, E, D and K) right out with it. By timing the dosages correctly, any loss of these vitamins will be minimal. Even if this timing advice were to be completely ignored, it would take about a year of incorrect use for any significant deficiency problem to occur. If you have any concerns, simply give your child a good multivitamin supplement each morning.

The only valid potential risk of mineral oil is inhalation by a child who is resistant to swallowing it. Explain to your child before-hand all the wonderful benefits of taking this "special medicine." If the child still refuses to cooperate, *you must not force it!* Inhaling mineral oil can cause a very resistant aspiration pneumonitis.[3] At the first sign of protest, stop the administration immediately. You will need to rely on fiber and dietary changes alone.

Part 2: Fiber

If used in sufficient quantity, fiber without mineral oil *may* be effective. However, it is not ideal and results will take longer. When I use the term "fiber," I am generally speaking of products containing psyllium husk, methylcellulose or inulin. Of these three, psyllium husk powders are the least expensive per dose. In recent years, companies began grinding the psyllium husk powder extra fine so most are no longer gritty or unpleasant. Psyllium husk powders come both plain and in a variety of flavors, both regular and sugar-free.

Methylcellulose is a soluble fiber product available as both a powder (for stirring into cold water) or as tablets. Products containing inulin, though a bit more expensive per dose, are probably the most acceptable to children. Inulin fiber comes in regular or sugar-free chewable orange-flavored wafers that taste as good as candy and has no grit. In fact, I would be surprised if any child didn't think they were getting a candy treat at each dose and ask you for more.

Whichever type of fiber you choose, I recommend initially starting off with at least double the highest recommended dose on the container. Divide this total amount into thirds, and give one-third three times a day. With each dose of fiber, urge fluids. Fiber works by taking the fluids you consume and holding them inside the colon. Increase the dose after each bowel movement until you are achieving the desired results, reducing the dose if stools become *too* loose.

Fiber is neither a laxative nor a medication, so there's no such thing as "overdosing." Fiber simply passes through the system, moving the stool along with it. The only possible consequence of too much fiber is loose stools—a far better scenario than the large, hard and impacted stools the child suffered with previously.

Consistency Is Key

During this initial period of determining the correct mineral oil and fiber dosing, be prepared for some stooling accidents. Despite every effort, a soft, lubricated stool is a lot more difficult to hold inside than a hard constipated stool. Eventually, your child will be physically unable to withhold, much to his or her dismay, and will likely have an accident. This is hardly grounds for punishment and *not* an appropriate time to enforce previous toilet training goals.

By following the mineral oil and fiber protocol faithfully, in combination as described, you will have created enough softness, bulk and lubrication to ensure relatively pain-free movements even if your child should succeed in withholding for several days in a row. The psychological factors will eventually recede, but only after the child has experienced enough pain-free movements firsthand. Day after day, week after week, month after month, the child will come to realize that it is once again safe to pass stool.

Even after things seem to have normalized, it is crucial to remain consistent with the protocol for quite some time because it only takes *one* recurrence of painful stool to jump-start the problem all over again. A lot depends on the child's personality, but I recommend continuing the mineral oil and fiber combination for about six additional months after the withholding stops in order to allow the psychological fear component to completely pass.

Once you are confident the vicious cycle is truly behind you, begin testing the waters by cutting the dose of *one* of these substances in half. About one month later, if all goes well, try cutting the dose of the other one in half. Continue cutting the dosages in this manner each month until the child is off both. Since neither are laxatives, any subsequent constipation would be due to dietary, exercise and/or psychological factors.

Kids and Food: Tough Love

In order to keep the bowels running smoothly, both adults and children also need regular exercise, adequate water intake and a healthy diet of natural Whole Foods. If I were raising a child today, I'd offer *only* Whole Foods in the most appealing kid-friendly varieties I could up with.[4] I'd also offer only water to drink, avoiding fruit juices altogether.

Parents often throw up their hands in resignation at the thought of getting their children to eat healthy, natural foods. Children are clever little beings who are experts at convincing their exhausted parents they would rather starve than eat vegetables, brown rice and other Whole Foods. Rather than engaging in a high-drama battle with the child, remain calm yet *firm*. There is no need to demand, threaten or force a child to eat a particular food or punish a child who refuses. Simply lead by example and continue to affirm, calmly and matter-of-factly, that the only two choices are to either eat what is being offered or be excused from the table.

No harm will come to even the most stubborn child who refuses to eat for several days. As long as parents remain firm, and the child *knows* the parents won't back down, the "battle" will pass rather quickly and the child will learn to enjoy the new foods. This aspect of "tough love" will pay off for the rest of the child's life. If new parents would attend to the correct dietary factors that prevent constipation, beginning at weaning, they could avoid ever having to deal with the nightmare of having a stool-withholding child.

As is the case with all chronic conditions in this book, the key to *permanent* reversal of constipation and stool withholding is to remove the causative factors that created them in the first place, and that includes following the 3LS Wellness guidelines outlined in Section IV of this book. In so doing, you will find any other chronic conditions and bothersome symptoms abating as well, and, you will also be preventing new health problems from occurring in the future.

CHAPTER 22

Excessive Body Odor

They always say time changes things,
but you actually have to change them yourself.

~ Andy Warhol
(American pop artist, 1928–1987)

Chronic Profuse Sweating

Chronic profuse sweating is an embarrassing problem to live with, and is, in fact, totally unnecessary. People suffering from this problem usually go to great lengths trying to hide it, slathering on antiperspirants, changing their clothes frequently and carrying handkerchiefs to continually blot the drips away. None of these approaches do anything to address the underlying cause of *why* you sweat far more than the average person: severe chronic stress-effect storage in the hypothalamus.

If trying to hide the fact that you're drenched in sweat weren't enough to deal with, you are probably also going to great lengths to hide or cover up the smell. In a healthy individual, sweat (in and of itself) has no unpleasant odor. It only stinks if you are sick, need metabolic detoxification or have poor hygiene habits. Even normal sweat will begin to stink after the bacteria living on the surface of your skin have had a chance to munch on the sweat and/or dead skin cells for awhile (due to infrequent showering or bathing). The bacteria then excrete waste products (bacteria poop) and *that's* the source of the offensive odor.

If your sweat stinks all the time, it is a pretty good indication that the bacterial population on your skin has become abnormally high. The solution is to rid yourself of the present (abnormal) bacterial population and then build another (normal) one from scratch. To get your bacteria count under control, simply shower twice a day with antibacterial soap for about three months. From that point on, usually once a day is enough for maintenance.

Care must be taken to avoid recontaminating your skin with the bacterial waste products present on your towels and clothing. Bacteria live and grow on dead organic matter, so when terry cloth towels and washcloths are *properly* used for drying (meaning, buffing off dead skin cells), bacteria naturally begin multiplying frantically on them. Bacteria also multiply on any sweat present on your clothing. Therefore, be sure to wash your towels, washcloths and clothing after each use during those initial three months. From that point on, a simple whiff of these items before use will easily let you know if the bacteria have been busy.

Body Odor Is Big Business

The entire body odor industry is thriving, with advertisements promoting the sales of antiperspirants, deodorants and body sprays everywhere you turn. These ads create the impression that not only are such products essential to resolving your "problem," but that normal sweat is undesirable, shameful and it also *stinks*! The ads never seem to point out that humans sweat all over their bodies, not just from the armpits. In fact, relative to the amount of sweat produced by the rest of the body, the percentage of perspiration emitted from the underarms is actually quite small.

If you, like most Americans, have bought into the mass assumption that antiperspirants are a safe and healthy way to combat body odor, read on. I stopped using antiperspirants over thirty years ago and encourage everyone to think twice before using them. Besides the fact that antiperspirants are not, and cannot ever be, a *cure* for sweating, there are several proven reasons behind my decision to abandon them.

Antiperspirants: Why I *Never* Use Them

First, antiperspirants contain aluminum, an ingredient now suspected to be directly related to Alzheimer's disease. More recently, the aluminum and paraben ingredients in antiperspirants have also been implicated as a possible contributing cause of breast cancer.[1] Second, I have seen continued use of antiperspirants cause permanent and devastating sebaceous cysts under the arms in certain individuals. ("Deodorants" without the antiperspirant component do not carry these risks.)

Antiperspirants are astringents that work by chemically puckering up the openings of the ducts of the sebaceous glands in the armpits. Antiperspirants attempt to hold the sweat *in*, which is completely unnatural to the body. Many people don't realize antiperspirants cannot actually stop the sweat glands from *making* the usual amount of sweat, only from *releasing* it. Thus, as soon as the antiperspirant either wears off or is washed away, your armpits will sweat even more profusely than before you put it on.

In some people, repeated and/or excessive use of antiperspirants can cause the sweat glands to eventually shut down and refuse to open at all. The sebum that is never allowed to exit the gland then builds up, causing sebaceous cysts. Once things have progressed to this unfortunate point, the ducts tend to be permanently damaged, and it is often too late to reverse the problem by simply stopping antiperspirant use.

I have assisted in surgical procedures in which patients have had to have the entire underarm skin area removed and new skin grafted, solely due to the formation of sebaceous cysts caused by repeated antiperspirant use. This crippling and deforming procedure is completely preventable. Why isn't there a warning on the product labels? Where is the FDA on this one?

If you have already developed one or more sebaceous cysts under your arms, pay attention to the warning. Stop using antiperspirants and try to save yourself from the nightmare just described by immediately starting moist, hot compresses for five minutes at a time, several times a day.* If you are lucky, your sweat glands might begin to believe you really want them to open back up. For some people, it may already be too late.

Any cysts that remain after two weeks of following the hot compresses protocol will likely need to be seen by a dermatologist for surgical removal. If you ever find yourself in this position, be sure to choose a skillful surgeon experienced in carefully removing *only* the individual glands that are damaged, because any neighboring normal ducts carelessly damaged during surgery could then require *additional* surgery.

---

* See Chapter 18: *Acne and Sebaceous Cysts* and Chapter 31: *Hot Compresses.*

Stinky Feet, Bad Breath and Excessive Gas

Of course, people are concerned with body odors of any kind, including the foul odors of stinky feet, bad breath and passing gas. Controlling foot odor can be more challenging than controlling general body odor because the feet continually perspire *and* shed a lot of dead skin. Yet have you ever wondered why some people have horribly stinky feet and others do not? Keeping the feet confined inside socks and shoes all day is one of the culprits; another is wearing shoes without socks.

Any perspiration or dead skin, whether on your terry cloth towels, on your socks, in your shoes or between your toes, really *stinks* when it rots. Wearing socks (which can be washed) prevents this dead skin and perspiration from getting inside your shoes (which are rarely if ever washed). People wouldn't dream of wearing the same socks for weeks, months or sometimes years at a time and expect their feet not to reek, so is it any wonder people who wear their shoes without socks have feet that stink so bad? Throw out any heavily contaminated shoes, and commit to a combination of wearing socks inside your shoes and going barefoot as much as possible.

Next, if you have chronic bad breath (halitosis), you've probably noticed you aren't having much success trying to "cure" the problem with breath mints, toothpaste, mouthwashes and tongue scrapers. This is because over 90% of the odor originates from the lungs, not from within the mouth itself. Foods such as onions and garlic, once digested, are absorbed into the bloodstream and carried to the lungs. You can verify this by noticing that the breath coming from your nose smells just as bad.

One form of halitosis known as "fecal breath" is usually a clear indication that the ileocecal valve (located between the large and small intestines) is incompetent. Rather than opening and closing when it's supposed to, it remains stuck open, allowing colonic sewage to be absorbed directly into the bloodstream. The body then attempts to eliminate these toxins through the lungs, causing the breath odor. Most chiropractors and massage therapists can teach you how to perform a self-massage technique that will improve ileocecal valve function.

While halitosis is almost always caused by leaky gut syndrome (LGS) and over-all system toxicity, a small percentage is caused by chronically diseased tonsils (from recurrent infection or allergies) that have lost the battle to bacteria. In permanently scarred tonsils, the tonsillar crypts (pockets) accumulate food particles, mucus and other debris. The immune system regards this debris as a foreign invader, sending white blood cells into the area, which create a putrid-smelling pus called tonsil stones or "tonsilloliths." This is called tonsillar cryptosis. Your doctor can make this diagnosis simply by pressing on the tonsil with an examining finger and expressing some of this whitish clumpy material. Such a diagnosis *may* warrant a tonsillectomy.

And finally, the brunt of much humor *and* embarrassment, "passing gas" is so common nearly everyone considers it "normal." But believe it or not, normal digestion produces no gas whatsoever. The only air in the gut should be what is swallowed with food or simply from nervous swallowing. Only the *fermentation* of undigested food causes gas. In fact, gas is a natural product of all fermentation. The old jokes about beans being the "musical fruit" are true. Beans contain raffinose, and since humans do not have raffinase (the enzyme that breaks down raffinose) in their guts, beans live up to their longstanding, well-deserved reputation.

Taking over-the-counter anti-gas preparations containing simethicone, when indicated, as well as including more soluble fiber in the diet and supplementing with probiotics can be helpful. Other over-the-counter products designed to prevent and/or alleviate excessive gas contain certain enzymes to assist in digestion. All such products can temporarily relieve gas, however leaky gut syndrome (LGS) and Candida-related syndrome (C-RS) are the main causes of abnormal enzyme production and must be addressed for long-term success.

Body Detoxification

A "toxin" can be defined as anything that is poisonous to the body, whether actively damaging or simply no longer useful. Toxic waste products originating from *outside* the body are called exotoxins, and toxic waste products produced *inside* the body are called endotoxins. Toxins tend to accumulate within the body until or unless they can be released.

Once processed by the liver and lymphatic system, the body has four pathways for ridding itself of toxins: stool (including gas), urine, breath and skin (including sweat and the shedding of dead skin cells). If any one of these channels is blocked, even partially, the others must take up the slack. If you want to get to the root cause of any body odor problem, *all* of these detoxification pathways must be considered.

Types of Toxins

- **Exotoxins:** Airborne pollution, heavy metals, chemicals such as chlorine, bromide and fluoride, pesticides, artificial ingredients, prescription drugs, alcohol, tobacco, etc.
- **Endotoxins:** Free radicals, uric acid, lactic acid, hormones no longer useful, ketone bodies from emergent fat metabolism, etc.

One of the quickest ways to clear and detoxify your system is through fasting. You could do a supervised water fast (meaning supervised by your trusted health practitioner), a juice fast using freshly made juices (especially vegetable), or various other types of fasts. If you are new to fasting, do some thorough research before you begin so you understand what you are trying to accomplish and how to do it safely.[2]

Fasting is an ancient and time-honored way of rejuvenating the body and the mind. Fasting is *not* starvation. With starvation, the person doesn't know whether they will ever get anything to eat again. The stress of that situation completely changes the body's hormonal response to the absence of food and causes accelerated damage. On the other hand, a person who is fasting knows they can eat at any time. This creates a totally different metabolic milieu, encouraging detoxification and causing health improvement.

There are many ways and means for assisting the detoxification pathways of the body, some of which include: adequate water intake, colonics or enemas, infra-red saunas, breathing exercises, Epsom salts baths, dry skin brushing, gentle rebounding, Rolfing and/or a massage series (three total-body deep-tissue therapeutic massages per week for two weeks in a row). Everything you do will work better if you simultaneously follow the 3LS Wellness protocol outlined in Section IV of this book. With the information in this chapter, you now understand how to overcome any embarrassing body odor issue while improving your over-all health and well-being at the same time.

Section IV

THE 3-LEGGED STOOL (3LS) OF WELLNESS

How to Prevent *and* Reverse Your
Chronic Health Conditions

CHAPTER 23

Introduction to the 3LS

As I see it, every day you do one of two things: build health or produce disease in yourself.

~ Adelle Davis
(American author and whole foods pioneer, 1904–1974)

Doing What It Takes

This section of the book will show you how to *do what it takes* to be healthy. It describes the three crucial lifestyle practices recommended throughout the first three sections. These are the most important guidelines I know of for improving health, preventing dis-ease and, to whatever degree possible, *reversing* chronic health conditions. I refer to them as the 3-Legged Stool of Wellness, or 3LS for short. The word Wellness along with its 3LS constituents—Skilled Relaxation (SR), Aerobic Exercise and Whole Foods— have been capitalized for emphasis throughout this book.

Each of the following three chapters will be devoted to one "leg" of the 3LS—providing all the information you need to successfully begin incorporating these life-changing practices into your daily routine. Although implementing even *one* leg of the 3LS can make a positive difference in your health, the fastest gains will be had by implementing *all three* legs simultaneously. Moreover, the benefits of doing more than one leg of the 3LS are not simply additive, they are *multiplicative*. For example, if one leg is worth 3 points, then combining two would be worth 9 points, and combining all three would be worth 27 points!

The Art of Prevention

By properly incorporating the 3LS of Wellness into your lifestyle, not only will you have the best chance for reversing any chronic health conditions you may already have—*at their root cause*—you will also learn how to prevent new health problems from developing in the future. This is as stated in Henry de Bracton's famous quote, "An ounce of prevention is worth a pound of cure." Since it is most often the absence of a Wellness lifestyle that causes dis-ease, logic follows that the 3LS protocol will give you the very best chance of preventing and reversing dis-ease. That goes for both chronic *and* acute health conditions.

The 3LS lifestyle practices described in this section work through improving homeodynamics, the greatest strength of the bodymind. One of the most amazing things about a holistic approach is that when you follow a lifestyle recommendation for one particular condition, many other symptoms or conditions tend to be healed or prevented at the same time. For example, the same underlying mechanism that is causing migraine headaches may also be causing arthritis, fatigue, irritable bowel and acne in the same patient.

> ***Health is an announcement of agreement between your body, mind and spirit.***
>
> ~ Neale Donald Walsch (1943)

The recent popular trend in the United States is to "go green," and not only for the environment. Out of sheer necessity, many of us are finally beginning to be more careful about what we choose to allow on, in and around our bodies, as well as in our homes. We are collectively beginning to pay attention to the importance of reducing the toxic burden of pesticides, chemicals, artificial sweeteners, electromagnetic radiation and so on. This coincides with the exciting new trend of becoming more aware of the role our thoughts, beliefs and emotions play in creating all aspects of life.[1]

We've come a long way since 2003, when a special issue of *Time* documented our new openness in this area of the mind-body connection. On its cover: "How Your Mind Can Heal Your Body." The bottom line today?

We are not helpless victims of dis-ease. Nor must we, as many of us have been led to believe, be at the mercy of the medical profession for our survival. The fact is, the majority of the healing process does not require a medical license. Nature tends to do an amazing job if we simply remove the factors that interfere with abundant health and become active participants in our own well-being.

The "Healing Crisis"

Keep in mind that, as you work toward Wellness, you may experience a phenomenon known as the "healing crisis." A healing crisis is a temporary worsening of symptoms, as well as a recurrence of symptoms that you may not have experienced for several years. Think of your health from birth to death as a train journey. When the train is reversed, health conditions that arose along the track of life will be temporarily revisited.

Many healing crisis issues are simply temporary withdrawal symptoms from the physical, mental and emotional addictions you have established with your former unhealthy lifestyle choices. Most healing crises come in cycles and are relatively short-lived. View these as positive signs that you are on the right track because when symptoms abate, you can look forward to enjoying a new, higher level of health.

One of the main purposes of this book is to help you understand that your choices are not limited to covering up your symptoms. The first step in preserving health and well-being is to *listen* to the messages and warnings your bodymind is trying to send you. Pay attention, and without allowing fear to call the shots, trust your own gut feelings. After all, who do you suppose knows your body most intimately—you or your doctor? Once you have read this book cover to cover a few times, having fully internalized all the information, you will have increased your chances of making informed decisions and decreased your chances of making decisions you could well regret for a lifetime.

Once you truly understand all your available options, you will have internalized all the information you need to fully commit to a plan of recovery. Before embarking on your healing journey, get a journal and write down the typical pattern of your conditions and symptoms. Notate their frequency, duration, severity and any other details you feel relevant.

Then, keep a journal or record over the next several months so you can clearly see the progress you are making along the way.

Wellness Works—Try It!

As a representative of holistic medicine, traveling and speaking throughout the country, I have learned that the most powerful influence on both physicians' and patients' attitudes about any new concept has always been *personal experience of results*.

By putting the 3LS principles into practice as described, within a matter of a few short weeks, you may find you no longer need to suppress your symptoms as much. Depending on how long you've been ill and how far advanced your dis-ease has progressed, you may even be able to look forward to a day when you are completely free of symptom-suppressing pharmaceuticals—a day when when you have moved *beyond disease care*! Remember: Always work with your physician to gradually reduce any medications no longer needed, and *never* discontinue any treatment without consultation and close supervision by the prescribing practitioner.

Imagine this: If only you so choose, you can be a walking, talking, living example of the power of a Wellness lifestyle. You can join the ranks of people who have firsthand experience of just how amazing it's possible to feel on an everyday basis. Then perhaps you, like myself, will feel compelled to *make your voice heard*. Demand change in how medicine is practiced—a change that will benefit us all now, as well as in the generations to come.

When it comes to creating abundant health, all the body's systems work together like an orchestra. Since the turn of the new millennium, the trend has finally been shifting back toward a renewed awareness of the innate intelligence of the body. Our bodies are some of the most remarkable things in creation, and when given proper support, they have the ability to heal themselves. To assist this natural process, we need only appreciate and be willing to incorporate the holistic lifestyle approaches described in the following three chapters. Wellness works—try it!*

---

* For more in-depth information on the 3LS, and *how* to successfully implement these practices into your lifestyle, see *Recapture Your Health,* co-authored by Walt Stoll, MD and Jan DeCourtney, CMT.

CHAPTER 24

Skilled Relaxation (The 1st Leg)

It's not that some people have willpower and some don't.
It's that some people are ready to change and others are not.

~ James Gordon, MD
(Founder of the Center for Mind-Body Medicine, 1991)

The "Relaxation Response"

Over the past four decades, Western medical science finally began taking notice of something many other cultures have known, honored and faithfully practiced for thousands of years. That "something" happens to be a particular state of mind which, when elicited on a regular basis through any one of a variety of techniques, has the ability to produce profound health benefits.

In 1975, Harvard Medical School doctor Herbert Benson, MD termed this special state of mind "The Relaxation Response" in his nationwide best-selling book by that name. He and other experts have come to the following consensus: The regular practice of *any* technique that produces the relaxation response in an individual has the potential to prevent or reverse nearly *every* chronic health condition imaginable.[1]

In Eastern cultures, the practice by which people reach this state of mind is called "meditation." Here in the West, some are uncomfortable with that term for personal or religious reasons and prefer to call it "relaxation" instead. Yet there is nothing inherently mystical or "new age" about this practiced state of mind. In fact, many of the world's most significant religions were founded by people who had discovered the validity of it for themselves.

No matter what you choose to call it, biofeedback instruments have determined that this meditative or relaxed state of mind involves nothing more than a preponderance of *alpha* or *theta* brain wave frequencies. The feeling is a calm, quiet sensation, very much like being on the verge of falling asleep. The greater the percentage of alpha and theta frequencies produced in the brain, and the higher their amplitude, the more profound the health benefits.

Because so many people today report finding it nearly impossible to "relax," many different tools and techniques exist for assistance in getting there. The only caveat is that there's no such thing as a single technique that works for everyone. What works for me may not work for you, and vice versa. I use the term "Skilled Relaxation" (SR) to denote the practice of any technique that brings about the relaxation response for *you*.

Once you have read through this chapter a few times and are ready to begin, keep in mind that, as the name implies, Skilled Relaxation is truly a *skill*. Like all skills, the more you practice, the better you will become at perfecting your favorite method(s). When practiced according to the guidelines in this chapter, you can look forward to every single system of your bodymind reaping the benefits. Even a partial list of the proven benefits that accrue from the regular practice of effective SR reads like a cure-all. Track your progress in a journal because it's easy to forget all the miserable symptoms you used to have once they begin to abate.

In addition to the long list of benefits provided on the following page, effective SR heals leaky gut syndrome (LGS) by allowing for the return of normal blood flow to the gastrointestinal tract (diverted due to living in a state of constant readiness). In this way, SR not only helps relieve local gastrointestinal distress symptoms directly related to LGS (such as constipation, diarrhea, cramps and indigestion) but more importantly, works toward relieving secondarily related neurological, endocrinological and immunological disorders.[3] I've received hundreds of testimonials over the years on my online bulletin board about the amazing benefits of SR. The only way I know of for you to begin to believe all these benefits are possible is to follow the guidelines in this chapter and experience them for yourself.

The *Amazing* Benefits of Skilled Relaxation[2]

- Lowers resting heart and respiratory rates
- Helps normalize weight (whether you are under or over-weight)
- Slows the aging process
- Normalizes blood pressure (both hypertension *and* hypotension)
- Lowers "bad" cholesterol levels and increases "good" blood fats
- Decreases fatigue
- Reduces insomnia
- Increases energy and productivity
- Strengthens the immune system
- Normalizes hormonal imbalances
- Prevents or reverses premenstrual syndrome (PMS)
- Prevents or reverses infertility
- Prevents or reverses chronic adult acne
- Alleviates chronic headaches
- Decreases or alleviates bodily aches and pains
- Increases mind-body coordination and physical agility
- Normalizes brain chemistry, benefiting mental and emotional health
- Relieves panic, anxiety, nervousness, phobias and neuroses
- Reduces drug dependency and various addictions
- Alleviates depression and psychosomatic illness
- Reduces feelings of inhibition, inadequacy and alienation
- Reduces irritability, anger and impatience
- Alleviates inner sense of hopelessness or meaninglessness
- Improves self-esteem and develops inner wholeness
- Increases autonomy and promotes self-actualization
- Improves problem-solving ability and organization of thinking
- Improves short-term memory ability and enhances creativity
- Expands one's ability to love and express affection

Brain Wave Frequencies

Quantum physics has demonstrated that all of creation is made up of waves of energy in motion, basically frequencies of vibration. Without any effort or awareness on your part, your brain (including your thoughts and emotions) are constantly producing various brain wave frequencies. The preponderance of these frequencies vary, primarily, depending on if you are wide awake, sound asleep or anywhere between the two. They also vary depending on your mental and emotional state.

Be the change you want to see in the world.

~ Mahatma Gandhi (1869–1948)

Scientists have broken these brain wave frequencies down into four groups and given each a name: *Beta* is the awake, thinking rhythm. Beta is represented by a preponderance of brain wave frequencies of 13 or more cycles per second (cps). *Alpha* (8–13 cps) and *theta* (4–8 cps) are states representing the progressive predominance of slower and slower primary brain wave frequencies that are the goal of SR. We all pass through alpha and theta frequencies before finally reaching *delta* (less than 4 cps), the state of sleep. Delta is also the point at which loss of muscle control occurs.

Brain Wave Frequencies

- **Beta** (13+ cps): Wide awake, alert, thinking state
- **Alpha** (8–13 cps): Relaxed concentration, light meditation
- **Theta** (4–8 cps): Deep relaxation, deep meditation
- **Delta** (below 4 cps): Sleep

As described in Section II of this book, our modernized society exposes most of us to more than 382,000 stressors every single day, 90% of which are environmental. Each individual stressor evokes the fight-or-flight (FOF) response to some degree, creating a state of *readiness*. All readiness not immediately released through the act of actually fighting or fleeing gets stored in the hypothalamus. Since the sheer volume of stressors we are exposed to daily are far beyond what can be discharged during a good night's sleep, this stored stress-effect builds up in increasing amounts daily from birth forward. People suffering from multiple chronic conditions often do not realize that, typically, *all* of their symptoms are related to this same basic mechanism.

Any form of SR that successfully gets your brain waves into alpha or theta automatically discharges the chronic build-up of stored stress-effect in your hypothalamus at a rate twenty-four times faster than normal sleep. In other words, twenty minutes of effective SR discharges the stress-effect equivalent of eight hours' worth of regular sleep! Given this advantage, within just 6–12 months of consistent twice-a-day practice, the average person will succeed in discharging the majority of their lifetime's worth of accumulated readiness. From that point on, once-a-day practice is usually sufficient for maintenance.

Finding and Certifying Your SR Technique

Visitors to my website often want me to tell them which SR technique is the "best," or they at least want me to recommend a few for them to try. The problem with that is, as I stated earlier, finding a method that works is an extremely individual process involving some trial and error. The thing to remember is, no matter which method you choose, if it fails to produce the relaxation response for *you*, it will fail to provide all the wonderful benefits ascribed to it. That being said, this chapter gives some suggestions that you may find helpful.

To begin with, I recommend obtaining a copy of *The Relaxation & Stress Reduction Workbook*.[4] This workbook provides a quick, easy and cost-effective way to learn some of the most popular SR techniques. Simply choose any technique that appeals to you and start experimenting. With a little perseverance, you will soon find one or two ways that fit your own personality and lifestyle, are easy and enjoyable to do, and will produce both immediate and long-term benefits. When you find a method that works for you, chances are you'll know (sense) it.

For producing the long-term health benefits listed in this chapter, timing is an important aspect to consider. Empirical observations have shown that the very *best* time of day to perform your first SR session is upon waking in the morning, *before* getting out of bed. If the thought of starting your day a little earlier sounds daunting, remember that each effective SR session gives you, in effect, the equivalent of the stress-reducing benefit of another eight hours' sleep. The second most beneficial time is immediately following exercise, and the third most beneficial time is two or more hours before going to sleep at night. The *worst* times (least effective for this purpose according to empirical observations) are right before exercising and less than one hour before going to sleep at night.

After the first 2–4 weeks of twice-a-day practice, once you are fairly certain you are consistently reaching the relaxation response, I highly recommend seeking out a biofeedback technician to verify scientifically that your SR technique is effectively producing alpha or theta frequencies in your brain. I call this "*certifying* your technique." In so doing, you won't run the risk of practicing for several months only to discover your efforts aren't actually paying off.

Obstacles: Falling Asleep and "Monkey Mind"

Throughout all my years of answering health questions on my website's bulletin board, I've become a bit of an expert on identifying the most common obstacles people encounter when they are new to the practice of SR. Not surprisingly, the most common problem of beginners is falling asleep, which unfortunately negates the session. Beginners often pass quickly from beta (the waking rhythm) all the way through to delta (the sleeping rhythm) because they haven't yet mastered enough control to maintain alpha and theta.

The best way to avoid falling asleep during SR is to sit upright with your spine erect, either in a chair with your feet flat on the ground or cross-legged on the floor or bed with hands resting comfortably on your lap. Avoid leaning your head against the chair or wall, which would again put you at risk of falling asleep. If you must lie down while performing SR, I recommend trying what I call the "Big Spoon Trick:" Hold a large spoon vertically in your hands atop your torso while performing SR. Since muscular control is lost the instant you slip past theta into delta (sleep), the spoon will drop from your hands and thump you awake so you can immediately return to your session without your efforts being wasted.

If you keep dropping off to sleep despite your best efforts, try not to get too frustrated. It shows you are at least on the right track and, with continued practice, you will soon learn enough control to stay in the correct frequency range without slipping over the edge into sleep.

Another challenge nearly every beginner has is something called "monkey mind." You're sitting quietly with the intention of doing an SR session, but your thoughts refuse to turn off. Your mind jumps from thought to thought in rapid succession and you feel powerless to make it stop. Remember what the masters say: "*This, too, shall pass.*" Even in everyday life, one of the hardest things to do is learn to release the constant chatter of the mind. Eckhart Tolle writes extensively about mind activity in his best-selling books.[5] He points out that mind chatter is due to a lack of presence—in other words, lamenting over the past and worrying about the future. The goal is to train your mind to be here, now, because *now is all there truly is.*

Getting frustrated by monkey mind will only make it worse. Instead of resisting or pushing against the stream of thoughts, just quietly and peacefully observe the thought without any attachment. Imagine each thought drifting or floating away from you, as if in a soap bubble. Be patient with yourself. It's not about trying to *make* the relaxation response happen. Instead, the idea is to learn to *let* it happen.

That being said, some people really are *so* overwhelmed with the bracing that results from overwhelming chronic stress-effect storage performing effective SR is virtually impossible. If this proves to be your experience, the easiest and least expensive option is to find a good massage therapist and get at least three 90-minute total-body deep-tissue therapeutic massages per week for two weeks in a row. This serves the purpose of manually discharging some of the built up stress-effect, thereby relieving much of the bracing that has been preventing you from successful SR practice. Since benefits of the massage series usually last only a few short months, take advantage of this time to perfect your SR technique.

Alternatives to the massage series include a full Rolfing series (once per week for ten weeks) or Hellerwork. Each would give benefits for about a year. Finally, I always recommend anyone afflicted with bracing to learn either Feldenkrais or the Alexander Technique and practice it regularly.[6]

Biofeedback and Entrainment

The same biofeedback machine used to certify your SR technique can also be used to help you learn how to reach the relaxation response in the first place. Biofeedback (meaning, feedback on your biology) simply monitors what the brain and body are doing. With this technological device, you can learn how different brain wave frequencies feel. You can also increase both awareness and control of your body's subtle physiological stress responses (heart rate, blood pressure, body temperature, etc.).

All of the techniques described in *The Relaxation & Stress Reduction Workbook* are "active" approaches—meaning you are the one putting yourself into the relaxed state. But external or "passive" means of reaching the relaxation response also exist. These involve various types of stimuli designed to *entrain* the brain to certain brain wave frequencies. Light and sound machines are in this category, as are certain types of audio CDs designed for this purpose (such as those containing a binaural beat).

Many people prefer a passive approach, especially in the beginning, because it allows them to be less concerned about learning techniques. Some even find the music or nature sounds in some recordings solves the monkey mind problem by providing a distraction from the constant stream of thoughts. The only possible risk with passive approaches is the *remote* chance of entrainment technologies precipitating a seizure in someone with known or borderline epilepsy. However, there is no such risk with any of the active approaches such as deep breathing, progressive relaxation, visualization and so forth.

In addition, I highly recommend experiencing group meditation. Due to our electromagnetic nature, a group of people practicing SR together will have an easier time reaching alpha or theta than an individual alone.[7] Even the crudest laboratory instruments have proven that we are each surrounded by a sixty-foot-wide ball of energy called an aura, and that aura is easily sensed by other nearby auras. When a group of people relax or meditate together, it is only natural (and therefore easier) to become attuned and entrained to this set of frequencies.

One final note: You don't have to believe in SR's effectiveness for it to work for you—you just have to do it! When it comes to the 3LS of Wellness (Skilled Relaxation, Aerobic Exercise and Whole Foods), SR is *by far* the leg that will bring the most significant long-term improvements in your health. Therefore, if you choose only one leg of the 3LS, let it be Skilled Relaxation.

CHAPTER 25

Aerobic Exercise (The 2nd Leg)

Action expresses priorities.

~ Mahatma Gandhi
(Political and spiritual leader of India, 1869–1948)

Why *Aerobic* Exercise?

There's no denying the importance of regular exercise for good health. Although *any* type of exercise is beneficial to the body, *Aerobic* Exercise provides many benefits that most other types of exercise cannot. Aerobic Exercise is the most effective type for cardiovascular health, the management of stress and the promotion of general health and well-being.[1]

So what, exactly, qualifies an exercise as "aerobic"? Aerobic Exercise is any type of non-strenuous, sustained exercise activity that 1) uses the large-muscle groups, 2) is rhythmic in nature, 3) gets your heart rate into what's known as the "target heart range" (THR) and then, 4) keeps your heart rate *consistently maintained* within that range for a minimum duration of 12½ minutes.

Aerobic Exercise is so named because it affects the way the body utilizes oxygen. During normal everyday activities, our bodies take in oxygen from the air we breathe and place it into storage for later use. During Aerobic Exercise, this stored oxygen is completely discharged, so the body must then immediately begin using oxygen directly from the air. The moment the body switches from using stored oxygen to using oxygen directly from the air is the moment the exercise becomes "aerobic." At that point, oxygen utilization becomes 15–25% more efficient.

Besides the obvious improvements you can expect to gain in strength, coordination and endurance, regular Aerobic Exercise helps normalize weight, whether you are overweight *or* underweight. It also builds up immune system reserves, normalizes blood pressure, helps prevent diabetes (and reduces insulin requirements in those who are already diabetic), lowers cholesterol levels, lowers the risk of various cancers, helps prevent osteoporosis and speeds the healing of injuries.

In addition to the physical benefits just mentioned, regular Aerobic Exercise also improves cognitive function and lowers the risk of dementia and Alzheimer's disease. It helps combat depression, anxiety and insomnia. And finally, regular Aerobic Exercise induces a positive mental outlook on life by increasing the production and release of the body's own natural endorphins (the "feel good" hormones).[2]

Some examples of activities that may qualify as "aerobic" (when performed at the proper individual intensity depending on your fitness level) include walking, jogging, stair stepping, jumping rope, lap swimming, cross-country skiing, bicycling, in-line skating, aerobic dance and chest-high water aerobics classes. Whichever exercise(s) you choose, it takes only three 20-minute sessions per week to reap all the wonderful benefits described in this chapter.

It's hard to believe something that takes so little time and is so easy (and fun) to do could produce so many benefits, but it *does!* You will never find a pill in a bottle that can even come close to doing what regular Aerobic Exercise does for your overall health and energy level. In fact, I know of very few valid excuses for *not* doing Aerobic Exercise. If you're too exhausted to even *think* about exercising, or feel you just can't find the time to fit exercise into your busy schedule, think again. Regular Aerobic Exercise is exactly what you need to get your energy back, thereby making everything else you do more efficient.

In fact, people who do regular Aerobic Exercise sleep more soundly, need fewer hours of sleep and awaken more refreshed than people who do not. They are also happier, more energetic and more productive overall. With a meager investment of your time, three times per week, the rewards will be returned to you many times over. The first step in beginning your exercise program is to determine your target heart range (THR).

Target Heart Range (THR)

Your THR is a heart rate range, in beats per minute, with the first number representing the lowest heart rate limit and the second number representing the highest heart rate limit. In order for your chosen activity to qualify as "aerobic," you must maintain your heart rate within this fairly narrow range throughout the duration (minimum of 12½ minutes) of exercise.*

Begin by calculating your maximum heart rate (MHR), which is the *maximum* number of times your heart should be able beat per minute. Your MHR number is 220 minus your age. For example, if you are 30 years old, your MHR would be 190 beats per minute. If you are 55 years old, your MHR would be 165. As you can see, your MHR decreases with age.

Now that you have determined your MHR, you can calculate your THR, which is between 60% and 80% of your MHR. Multiply your MHR by .60 for the lowest number in the range, and again by .80 for the highest number in the range. The following chart gives examples of the MHR and THR at ages 20, 35 and 60.

Examples of Target Heart Ranges

Age 20	Age 35	Age 60
MHR: 220 − 20 = 200	MHR: 220 − 35 = 185	MHR: 220 − 60 = 160
60%: 200 x .60 = 120	60%: 185 x .60 = 111	60%: 160 x .60 = 96
80%: 200 x .80 = 160	80%: 185 x .80 = 148	80%: 165 x .80 = 128
THR: 120–160	**THR: 111–148**	**THR: 96–128**

* Before beginning any type of Aerobic Exercise activity other than walking, check with your doctor to see if you need a stress test. If you have heart disease or are already at risk for an imminent coronary, your target heart range (THR) will be different than the standard formula described in this chapter.

The goal of any successful Aerobic Exercise session is to first *get* the heart rate into your THR, and then *keep* the heart rate consistently maintained within that range for the duration of the exercise (minimum 12½ minutes).[3] No matter which activity is chosen, in order for it to qualify as "aerobic," you must exercise at whatever intensity accomplishes those objectives. The intensity needed for *you* will depend on your current fitness level. If you are obese or have been sedentary for a long period of time, you may reach your THR doing nothing more than carefully marching in place, or taking a slow walk while gently swinging your arms. In general, the more fit and active you are, the more exercise intensity it takes to reach your THR. For one individual, walking slowly on a treadmill or pedaling slowly on an exercise bike is enough. For another individual, getting the same cardiovascular effect may require running, stair stepping or jumping rope.

Although full benefits of Aerobic Exercise are had in as little as 12½ minutes of sustained activity within your THR, it usually takes several minutes for the heart rate to reach the lowest limit in that range. Therefore, as a general rule, I recommend performing the exercise consistently for 20 minutes to ensure you have maintained your THR for that minimum 12½ minutes. Remember, the THR must be maintained *consistently* for the entire duration of exercise, so do not stop and re-start the activity at any time except to do a quick check of your pulse rate.

Heart Rate Check: The Six-Second Count

To verify you have reached and are exercising within your THR, you will want to perform a heart rate check after the first five minutes or so of activity. Many modern treadmills and other aerobic equipment have automatic heart rate monitors. If yours does not, or if you have chosen a different type of exercise, you will need to check it manually. Locate one of your pulse points, either on the wrist (radial) or neck (carotid), while having visual access to a clock or watch that displays seconds.

Although a fifteen-second count may be a bit more accurate, I find a six-second count to be the most convenient for two reasons. First, you can simply add a zero to the number you counted. For example, if you count 14 beats in six seconds, your heart rate is about 140 beats/minute.

Second, a six-second count will allow you to get back to your exercise faster. As soon as exercise stops, the heart rate normally slows rapidly. The longer you pause to take your pulse, the more risk you run of falling out of your THR. Pause just long enough for the six-second count, then immediately return to your exercise. With the six-second count, there is virtually no math involved and virtually no risk of your heart rate dropping below your THR during the count.

In addition to the first pulse check at the five-minute mark, re-check your heart rate anytime you feel you may be working too hard or not hard enough. With experience, you will develop a sense of your pulse rate and lessen the need for frequent checking.

A defining feature of Aerobic Exercise is that it should *never* be exhausting—no matter which type of activity you choose. Done correctly, you will have more energy after the activity than you had before you began. If you are huffing and puffing and drenching your clothes with sweat, chances are you are exceeding your THR. Working beyond the limits of your THR is considered *anaerobic* exercise, which falls under a completely different category and will not provide the benefits described in this chapter.

Injuries Defeat the Purpose

Chapter 6 described the fight-or-flight (FOF) response and "bracing" (total-body chronic muscle tension), along with its connection to accumulated stored stress-effect in the hypothalamus. Aerobic Exercise naturally discharges some of this bracing because the physical activity itself is so similar to fighting or fleeing.

The chronic muscle tension of prolonged bracing causes significant wear and tear on the skeletal system. When muscles are too tight, opposing muscle groups end up working against one another, creating a high risk of injury. Of course, any injury that puts you out of commission defeats the whole purpose of your exercise goal. Therefore, if your muscles are tense and tight, I recommend either the massage series previously described (three 90-minute total-body deep-tissue therapeutic massages per week for two weeks in a row), Rolfing or Hellerwork before you even *think* about doing any exercise other than walking.[4]

After addressing any severe bracing and obtaining clearance from your doctor, you are ready to begin a regular Aerobic Exercise regimen of 20 minutes, three times per week. Before you begin, determine your pre-fitness resting heart rate (RHR) by taking your pulse when you are completely at rest, such as before getting out of bed in the morning. People with a fit cardiovascular system tend to have lower RHRs. You will find that within 4–6 weeks of regular Aerobic Exercise, your RHR will have dropped about 15–25%. The drop in RHR is a direct measure not only of the discharge of accumulated stress-effect storage but also your increased metabolic efficiency *and* your decreased rate of aging.

Non-Aerobic Exercise

Aerobic Exercise is the main focus of this chapter because it provides the most comprehensive benefits for the purposes of the 3LS of Wellness. However, several types of non-aerobic exercise are also well worth mentioning. The list on the following page briefly describes the most important purpose and/or effects of each.

No matter what type(s) of exercise you select, check with your doctor before beginning. If the thought of taking on a regular exercise program seems insurmountable, just take it one day at a time. You might be surprised how quickly you progress. Go slow and easy at first, listening carefully to your bodymind as you progress. Within a few short weeks, you will already have experienced some noticeable benefits that will motivate you to continue. You may even find yourself actually enjoying and looking forward to your workouts. Within a month, you will likely notice a *significant* improvement in your over-all health and sense of well-being.

Types of Non-Aerobic Exercise

- **Gentle Stretching:** Helps improve flexibility, alleviating the discomforts of aging as well as symptoms of arthritis, fibromyalgia (FMS) and chronic fatigue syndrome (CFS).
- **Gentle Walking:** Although moderate to fast-paced walking falls into the category of Aerobic Exercise for many individuals, gentle walking is excellent for general metabolic health and is a good starting point for anyone not yet able to participate in other types of activity.
- **Rebounding:** Stimulates lymph circulation, which greatly assists detoxification processes.
- **Resistance Training:** Also known as weight training, this type of activity builds and maintains muscle and bone mass, increases strength and decreases body fat by increasing metabolism.
- **Isometrics:** Ideal for the goal of building muscle mass quickly.
- **Underwater Exercise (chest-high):** Ideal for those with generalized arthritis or localized conditions of the knees, hips, ankles or feet that make weight bearing undesirable.
- **Tai Chi, Qi Gong, Yoga and other gentle Eastern disciplines:** Ideal for relaxation, spiritual awareness and general health and well-being. For some individuals, these disciplines can also serve as an effective form of Skilled Relaxation (SR).

CHAPTER 26

Whole Foods (The 3rd Leg)

Leave your drugs in the chemist's pot
if you can heal the patient with food.

~ Hippocrates
(Greek physician, 400 BC)

What Are "Whole Foods"?

"Whole Foods"—if you're not quite sure what this means, you're not alone. The term has become such an integral part of my everyday vocabulary that I tend to forget it's still foreign to many. That is, until someone gives me that perplexed look and asks, "Whole what? Which kind of foods?" I guess such a response shouldn't be too surprising since the disaster that is today's standard American diet (SAD) consists almost entirely of *refined* foods, not Whole Foods. We have become a society that eats whatever is cheap, quickly available, requires little or no preparation and gives us the biggest flavor rush possible.

Simply stated, Whole Foods are those foods that are in their natural state, the way nature created and intended them. Some examples include fresh or frozen vegetables, fresh or frozen fruits, brown rice, nuts and seeds, 100% whole grains, unpeeled potatoes, dried beans, free range unprocessed lean meats, free range eggs, natural cheeses, real butter and pure clean water. In other words, Whole Foods are what we human beings were designed to eat—and did eat—before methods were invented to alter and refine our food supply.

Of course, you won't find many natural, unprocessed selections at your local fast food drive-thru. Even the majority of our grocery store aisles are stocked with processed "convenience" foods in cans, jars and boxes. Only around the perimeter of the store do you typically find Whole Foods.

The story of how we started refining our food supply began with food manufacturers' attempts to extend shelf life. Since no self-respecting pest or fungus will eat what's inside our canned and boxed packages (unless they have no other choice), these refined products can sit on the store shelf for weeks, months or even years. A long shelf life may be wonderful for the profits of the food industry, but not so wonderful for the health of the human body.

Even though we humans *are* highly evolved, our physiology has not yet adapted to refined foods as a dietary staple. Unlike with fungi and bugs who perish quickly, it can take months, years or even decades for damage to our bodies to even *begin* to become evident. How soon that damage begins to appear, and what form of dis-ease it takes, depends on each individual's genotype (genetic makeup) as well as the various lifestyle choices we make every single day.

Prior to the Industrial Revolution, refined foods did not even *exist* for the general public's consumption. Sugar was available only as a luxury, or via the pharmacy to "help the medicine go down." The National Research Council's recommended daily allowance of sugars and refined carbohydrates is zero—zilch! The fact that *any* amount of refined carbohydrate in the diet reduces health has been known by the government since it was first studied over a century ago.[1]

Refined Carbohydrates: The Opposite of Nutrition

Not all carbohydrates ("carbs") are created equal. A natural, *complex* carbohydrate contains, within itself as a living food, all the exact proportions of vitamins, minerals, proteins, enzymes and fiber necessary for its own metabolism. There are literally hundreds of micronutrients our bodies need for perfect health. Most of these essential nutrients are contained within the coating, peeling and/or germ—the very parts that are stripped, separated and removed from the original food during the refining process at the manufacturing plant.

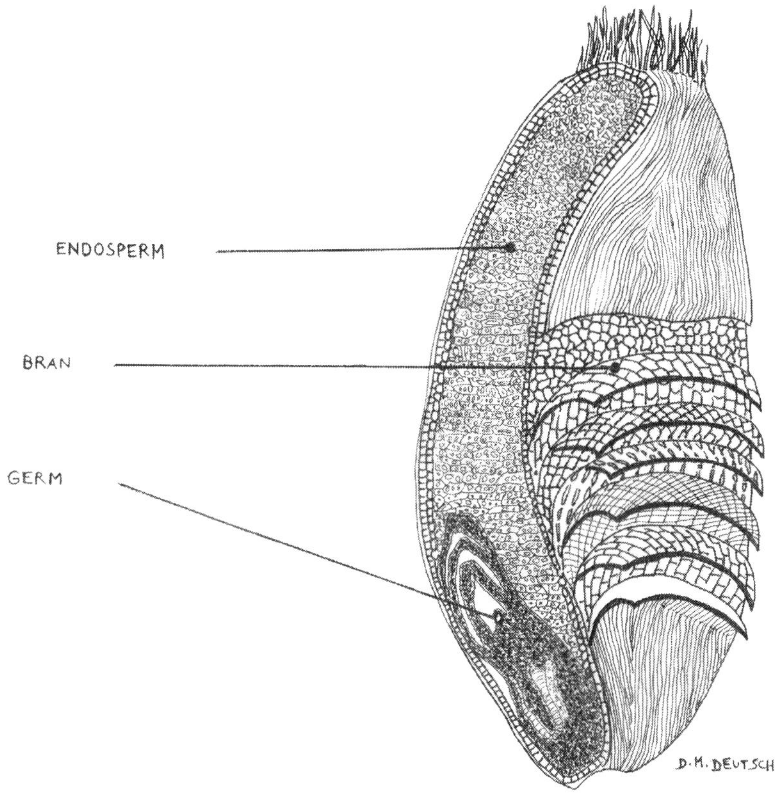

Whole Wheat Grain

An unstripped wheat grain is whole; refined wheat (white flour) is not. Brown rice is whole; white rice is not. Fresh and frozen fruits and vegetables are whole; fruit juice, canned fruit and canned vegetables are not. Each time you eat these and other *refined* carbohydrates, your body must immediately provide (somehow from somewhere—anyone have a magic hat?) all the essential substances manufacturing has removed, just to be able to *metabolize* that carbohydrate. In nearly all cases it cannot, and a chronic deficiency is created. Sounds like the opposite of nutrition, doesn't it? It truly *is*.

After stripping away more than a hundred documented essential nutrients during the refining process, manufacturers artificially replace about ten of them back into the new, refined product, then label it "enriched"—leading an unsuspecting public into believing they are buying (and eating) health-promoting foods. Nothing could be further from the truth! Even worse, the artificially replaced nutrients are being re-added according to outdated recommended daily allowance (U.S. RDA) standards, long known to be ridiculously low. People who regularly eat refined carbohydrates are likely to be seriously deficient in at *least* vitamins C, E and B complex, as well as the minerals magnesium, zinc and calcium.* These particular vitamins and minerals also happen to be the ones most depleted by stress.[2]

Aside from what the manufacturer's refining process does to grains such as wheat and rice, you would do well to avoid similar actions with your Whole Foods at home. An unpeeled potato, carrot or apple is whole; a peeled one is not. Eating an apple or a potato (even baked or mashed) without eating all the skin it was grown in creates the same refined carbohydrate deficiency situation just described. Of course, not all types of peeling are meant for consumption (banana peels, orange peels, nut shells, egg shells, etc.).

The damaging effects of refined carbohydrates reach far beyond simply being "empty calories." Refined carbohydrates cause more stress to the human body than all the other nutritional stresses combined.[3] On top of the induced deficiency of many vitamins, trace minerals and essential fatty acids (EFAs), our bodyminds have the added stress of trying to cope with additional insults such as chemicals, hormones, irradiation and now, genetic engineering.

Dennis Burkitt, MD (after whom Burkitt's lymphoma was named) wrote about the health effects of a refined carbohydrate, low-fiber diet back in the 1950s, where he spent many years in Africa as a medical missionary. He noted that whenever a patient came in with acute abdominal pain, he could rule appendicitis either in or out by the patient's answer to the following: "Do you eat the traditional diet of your ancestors or do you

* The U.S. government is slowly leaving behind the old RDA standards in favor of newer ODA (optimal daily allowance) standards. Nutritionally speaking, the best approach is to begin eating Whole Foods very early in life. For those who didn't start young, taking a high-quality nutritional supplement is a great way to catch up.

eat the white man's diet?" Dr. Burkitt reported never having found a case of appendicitis in patients still eating their natural ancestral diet.

Sugars and refined carbohydrates also depress the immune system, resulting in frequent and/or chronic illness.* Several mechanisms combine to explain the immune-depressing effect of sugars, the most important being the *leukocytic index*. The immune system's white blood cells, called leukocytes, protect us from invading organisms. The leukocytic index is a measure of how many pathogenic (disease causing) organisms one leukocyte can eat in one hour. A leukocytic index of 10 would indicate that one leukocyte ate ten organisms in that particular hour. The average leukocytic index in the United States is about 13.9. Diabetics generally have an average leukocytic index of less than 2.

Within fifteen minutes of ingesting the amount of refined carbohydrates found in the typical American evening meal (about 100 grams), the leukocytic index drops to an average of about 1.4—even lower than that of a diabetic.[4] Your own post-meal number may be higher or lower than this average, depending on your genetic makeup. A drop from 13.9 to 1.4 indicates a loss of over 90% of immune function immediately after indulging. This deficiency lasts for about two hours after each ingestion.

Obesity: *Not* the Only Consequence!

Before continuing, one clarification: When I use the word "diet" in this chapter, I'm not referring to a fad or short-term plan, such as "going on a diet" to lose weight. Instead, I use the term "diet" to denote a healthful way of eating with the intention of evolving it into a life-long habit.

The media focuses on the obesity epidemic as if putting on a few extra pounds were the only consequence of a poor diet. We are led to believe that our main concern should be counting calories and fat grams, not whether it is healthful to eat processed, refined, artificially sweetened products in the first place. Just because obesity is reflected physically in the mirror doesn't mean it is the only condition caused by poor diet.

* Given this knowledge, the common practice of giving glucose (sugar) water through intravenous drip to patients in hospitals makes no sense whatsoever. In fact, when Ringer's lactate (an intravenous solution containing no sugars) is given during and after surgery in place of the usual glucose water, there is a two-thirds reduction in post-operative infection.[5]

In reality, there are countless thin or normal-weight people (who may look perfectly fine on the outside) suffering from multiple chronic health conditions.

Just for a moment, throw away all preconceptions about what constitutes a "normal" diet—meaning, forget what you see everyone around you eating on a daily basis. Then, ask yourself the following: Was the human body really designed to eat a diet that defies what nature and the earth originally had to offer? What might be the eventual consequences of eating heavily altered foods with nearly all their micronutrients removed? What health effects might you anticipate from a lifetime of eating foods with added chemicals, preservatives and other unnatural ingredients you can hardly even pronounce? Are you more careful about what you feed your dog than you are about what you feed yourself? Would you attempt to fuel your car with something other than that which it was originally designed to operate on? If you did, would you expect your car to run smoothly, without various system breakdowns, and to last for several years to come? What are *you* eating day in and day out? What are you feeding your children?

All human actions have one or more of these seven causes: chance, nature, compulsion, habit, reason, passion and desire.

~ Aristotle (384 BC–322 BC)

Individuals raised on diets heavy in refined carbohydrates usually have no frame of reference for how amazing they could feel by eating Whole Foods according to the guidelines provided in this chapter. Many of today's youth eat a diet that is almost completely devoid of Whole Foods, feasting almost exclusively on fast food and processed, refined, high fat, high sugar, artificially-flavored versions. Even our nation's school lunch programs are serving up pizza, chicken nuggets, french fries and chocolate milk as a daily staple.

If you've never been a fan of vegetables and other healthy options, take heart. A refined carbohydrate diet numbs out the taste buds. There are hundreds of great tastes out there you may never have experienced simply because you have been trading that one taste, *sweet*, for all the rest. After the first few weeks, your new natural Whole Foods really *do* begin to taste amazingly good. Think of this as an exciting discovery of new taste adventures. Soon, you will get over the need for artificial appetite stimulants and the taste-bud numbing effect of your old diet. Don't be surprised if you soon find yourself repulsed by the thought of the heavy, processed, super-sweet foods you used to crave.

The difference between simply eating more Whole Foods and embarking on a *perfect* Whole Foods diet (PWFD) is that the latter involves the complete and total elimination of *all traces* of refined carbohydrates. After reading the following, you can decide whether you are willing, and ready, to embark on the PWFD.

"Perfect" Whole Foods?

Many people have no idea that refined carbohydrates (such as white flour, white rice and peeled potatoes) cause the exact same immunological reactions in the body as pure sugar. These reactions are related to the complex mechanisms of the Krebs cycle (how living cells convert food to energy), the full understanding of which goes beyond the scope of this book. For our purposes, suffice it to say that refined carbohydrates set up an *addictive* process in the bodymind, which explains the high failure rate when people attempt to switch to a more natural diet. Addiction to refined carbohydrates (including "junk foods") creates a vicious cycle in which "continued use of the addictive substance induces adaptive changes in the brain that lead to tolerance, physical dependence, uncontrollable craving and, all too often, relapse."[6]

Some people are willing to improve their diets, but are reluctant to attempt a *perfect* Whole Foods diet. Although it is true that *any* move toward Whole Foods (and away from refined foods) is beneficial, only the perfect diet will allow you to overcome the addictive aspect. It usually boils down to how badly you want to feel better. Since the thought of a potential life-long, drastic dietary change is admittedly too overwhelming for most, I encourage people to begin like I did, by committing to a two-week trial. By the end of the second week, most people are so impressed by the benefits, they find more than enough motivation to keep going.

When and if you decide to take the plunge and embark on the perfect diet, not only will you experience startling benefits within the first two weeks, you can also expect to see additional incredible health improvements *on a weekly basis* for the next 3–6 months.* After that point, as the rest of this chapter will explain, your immune system will have overcome the addictive aspect of refined carbohydrates and your bodymind will have stabilized at a new, healthier level of functioning not previously possible.[7]

Unless you're willing to eat only brown rice and vegetables as I did when I first started, I see little chance you could follow a perfect diet without all the facts. Refined carbohydrates are literally lurking everywhere, under many disguises. Before you begin, I recommend obtaining a copy of *The Healing Power of Whole Foods* by Beth Loiselle.[8] Beth's book is comprehensive, containing three quick reference sections in the back for looking up foods, additives and even brand names. The first edition of her book allowed fruit on the diet, but a correction has been made in the second edition. Fruits are high in natural sugar in proportion to their micronutrients, so have the potential to prolong your initial withdrawal phase. For this reason, I recommend eliminating all fruits for *at least* the first two weeks.

It's relatively easy to identify the more obvious sources of refined carbohydrates out there, such as sugar, brown sugar, high-fructose corn syrup, honey, molasses and fruit juice. Less obvious sources include sorbitol, mannitol and any word ending with "ose," such as sucrose, dextrose, lactose and fructose. (Note: This is *not* an all-inclusive list). Finding and eliminating all traces of refined carbohydrates takes education, research and diligent attention, which is why Beth's book is such an invaluable resource.

Hidden sugars abound. For example, many medications and supplements have forms of sugars added as binders or fillers (not all of which are clearly listed on the labels). Even iodized table salt has dextrose (a sugar) added to it as a stabilizer for the iodide. Alcohol is the most

---

* Note to diabetics and hypoglycemics: Be sure to consult your doctor before you begin. Your insulin or hypoglycemic medication requirements will be greatly reduced and you will need close professional supervision to monitor your progress. If you are like many individuals who follow the perfect Whole Foods diet, you may even reach a point where you are off all medications and are no longer considered a diabetic or hypoglycemic patient.

refined of all carbohydrates. Caffeine—a stimulant drug found in coffee, tea, cola and chocolate—fools the body into thinking it has eaten sugar. The amount of caffeine present in one large cup of coffee releases the equivalent of seven teaspoons of pure sugar from the liver into the blood. Even decaffeinated coffee contains some caffeine. Whole wheat flour should be considered refined unless it says "100% whole grain." These are just *some* examples of why education is important. For a proper trial, you must identify and eliminate *all* such items containing traces of refined carbohydrates, and be prepared to endure some withdrawal.

Withdrawal: What to Expect

A defining characteristic of *all* addiction (nicotine, alcohol, caffeine, drugs, etc.) is the presence of withdrawal symptoms upon elimination of the offending substance. Switching from refined foods to Whole Foods is no exception. If there is no addiction, there can be no withdrawal! When it comes to refined carbohydrate addiction, withdrawal symptoms tend to manifest as accentuated versions of the various symptoms you are already experiencing in your day-to-day life (typically as a result of your current diet).

Common withdrawal symptoms include headaches, fatigue, drowsiness, intense cravings, mood swings, weakness, trembling, chills, anxiety, nervousness, nausea, vomiting, dizziness, mental confusion, visual disturbances and more. Sounds a lot like what a drug addict might endure during withdrawal, doesn't it? In fact, an addiction to refined carbohydrates really *can* be as powerful as an addiction to hard-core drugs. The December 2008 edition of *Discover* featured an article entitled "Move Over, Heroin: 'Sugar Addiction' May Be a Reality."[9] Where are all the inpatient detox centers for this pervasive problem?

Typically, the more severe your withdrawal symptoms, the more severe the addiction. Likewise, the more severe the addiction, the more you stand to gain by *overcoming* the addiction. Strong withdrawal symptoms are proof positive of the extreme degree to which your unhealthy diet has been affecting your health all these years. Once refined carbohydrates are fully out of your system, you can expect rapid and exciting health improvements. The most important thing (which cannot be emphasized enough) is to be certain your elimination of refined carbohydrates is *perfect*—allow no traces.[10]

Total Avoidance Means *No Traces*

Sneaking tiny tastes of forbidden foods here and there will only sabotage your efforts, inducing strong cravings and prolonging your withdrawal symptoms indefinitely. You simply *cannot* succeed in breaking the addictive cycle of refined carbohydrates unless you are as diligent in your elimination as a person with a life-threatening peanut allergy has to be with avoiding all possible traces of the peanut protein (including potential cross-contaminations) every single day.

Although getting through the withdrawal phase can admittedly be challenging, the symptoms will pass in an average of 3–4 days. By the fifth day, you will be feeling much better and can move on to your second objective—reaching the two-week marker—at which point your cravings will have subsided and you will feel significantly better than you have in a long time, if not your entire life. The benefits will be *undeniable*. Then, it takes an average of an additional 3–6 months to reach your bodymind's ultimate objective: "forgetting" it was ever addicted to refined carbohydrates in the first place.

Three Objectives of the PWFD

1. Get through the initial withdrawal phase (average of 3½ days).
2. Move beyond the cravings and reach the point where the real benefits become obvious (average of 2 weeks).
3. Reach the point where the bodymind "forgets" the addiction (average of 3–6 months).

Fully understanding *how* to do the PWFD correctly, as well as *why* it must be done perfectly, will give you the greatest chance of success. Be sure to line up a support system before you begin. Create a two-week calendar so you can cross off each day as you go along. Obtain a journal so you can write about what you notice physically, mentally and emotionally. Make a list of your current symptoms and post it in the kitchen to remind yourself of why you are making this choice. Keep your goal firmly in mind at all times, knowing that the rewards will be greater than you could ever have imagined.

With Beth Loiselle's book in hand, and once you have familiarized yourself with its contents, you'll embark on "day 1." If you work weekdays, begin the diet on a Thursday morning because the full force of your withdrawal symptoms won't likely kick in until Friday afternoon. You'll be able to get through the worst of it relaxing at home over the weekend. By Monday morning you will have significant relief, and from there it only gets better. By the end of the second week, most people are shouting from the rooftops about how great they feel (and they have only just *begun* to see the benefits!).

Prolonged withdrawal symptoms (beyond the first week) is a sure sign you are still eating traces of something refined. Usually, this scenario is due to a gap in understanding of the ins and outs of everything that must be eliminated. Read every label, including those of any supplements and medications you may be taking, and bring Beth's book with you every time you shop. Without this resource, you could be sabotaging your success without even knowing the culprits.

Since the whole purpose of making the effort to conduct a two-week therapeutic trial is to experience what life can be like on a perfect diet (after withdrawal symptoms have passed), *any* slip up, intentional or accidental, defeats that purpose. Cheating will only make you highly symptomatic, falsely leading you to believe the perfect diet won't work for you. It *will*, if you follow it correctly.

Stick with It: Permanent Benefits in 3–6 Months

After the first two weeks of total elimination, you will enter the next phase, during which your system will become *hypersensitive* to refined carbohydrates, even in trace amounts. In other words, if you attempt to return to old ways of eating at this point, you will have an unpleasant reaction—a loud and clear message from your bodymind. One sip of an old favorite soda or a few bites of a saltine cracker will leave you feeling miserable and place you back into the withdrawal phase.

Based on my many years of experience with patients as well as assisting individuals via my online message board, I have learned that it takes anywhere from 3–6 months of maintaining the perfect diet for the body to literally *forget* it was ever addicted, at which point most people can tolerate a more liberal Whole Foods diet *without* triggering the addiction-withdrawal cycle. About 25% of people (the lucky ones) reach that goal in only three months. Since nearly 100% of people reach that goal by the end of six months, that is my recommendation. Any cheating or accidental slip-up with the diet before the happy day when the immune system resets will send you back to square one as far as the addictive process goes. To explain how the immune system resets, I will use the tetanus booster as an analogy.

We immunize children against tetanus by giving the antigen (vaccination) every month for three months, followed by a booster one year later. After this initial series, a booster is only needed once every ten years to maintain immunity. Nearly everyone's system "remembers" how to make the antibody against the tetanus antigen for at least ten years at a time, meaning the immune response is retained for that period of time. If a tetanus booster is not given for say, fifteen years, the body may have "forgotten" how to make the antibody and the entire tetanus immunization process would have to be repeated from scratch.

In the same way a tetanus booster can provide that *desirable* immune response for about ten years, a trace of refined carbohydrate can provide that *undesirable* immune response for about 3–6 months. The immunological process is the same, except luckily it takes far less time for the body to forget how to make the antibody for refined carbohydrates than it takes it to forget the antibody for tetanus. Doing the diet incorrectly (slipping up here, cheating a little there) keeps the antibodies at their peak memory and will only lead to perpetuation of miserable withdrawal symptoms and endless cravings, as well as both physical and emotional stress.

In my point of view, six months is a relatively short period of time to invest when the rewards to your health and energy levels are so great. You'll never know until or unless you do it! Obviously, a perfect Whole Foods diet takes significant planning and effort, especially in the beginning. Gone are the days of stopping at the deli or drive-thru window during lunch hour or on your way home from work. If it were not for the amazing short-term benefits of the first two objectives, few people would have enough motivation to stick with the diet long enough to get the long-term benefits of the third.

At the end of six months, you may wish to conduct a "test" to verify you've reached the third objective. Testing is done by eating a very *small* amount of refined carbohydrate. If you experience no unpleasant symptoms, congratulations! You have accomplished your long-term goal and can now handle small amounts of refined carbohydrates without experiencing a reaction. The closer you are to the six-month point of being perfect with the diet, the better your chances that your body has forgotten the addiction.

Since there is no way of knowing whether you are among the lucky 25% who will reach the third objective in only three months, it's risky to test before the six-month point. If your test induces symptoms, you may be back to square one as far as accomplishing your long-term goal (remember the tetanus booster analogy). The good news is that, either way, your efforts have *still* greatly improved your health in more ways than you can count on both hands.

Section V

HOLISTIC TOOLS

Safe and Effective
Alternative Therapies

CHAPTER 27

Elimination/Provocation Diet

The doctor of the future will give no medicine,
but will interest his patient in the care of the human frame, in diet,
and in the cause and prevention of disease.

~ Thomas Alva Edison
(American inventor and scientist, 1847–1931)

Multiple Symptoms: Which Way Is Up?

If you've flipped ahead to this chapter, chances are something you read earlier in this book caused you to suspect you may have hidden food hypersensitivities contributing to your symptoms and affecting your quality of life. Unlike "classic" food allergies, which most people associate with sudden and unmistakable (even life-threatening) reactions, food hypersensitivities tend to be much more vague and difficult to discern. Food hypersensitivities can mimic just about every symptom you can think of—fatigue, mood swings, brain fog, anxiety, cravings, chronic congestion, chronic pain, skin problems, heart palpitations, excessive sweating and so on.*

With multiple and/or vague symptoms manifesting in such unpredictable patterns, many people find themselves going from doctor to doctor only to be told all their tests have come back "normal." Yet how can you enjoy life when you feel fine and energetic one hour or day, then exhausted and miserable the next? You're not even sure "which way is up" anymore. Whenever patients describe this type of scenario, I'm almost

* See Chapter 9: *Allergy and Hypersensitivity* and Chapter 26: *Whole Foods.*

certain hidden food hypersensitivities are a main contributing factor. Since no one can have this problem without first having at least some degree of leaky gut syndrome (LGS), and since an estimated 75% of the population in the United States falls into this category, my suspicion is usually valid.

The question you may be asking yourself is: How do I find out for sure which foods I might be reacting to? Rather than subjecting yourself to conventional allergy tests which are capable only of detecting *serum* sensitivities (classical allergies) and not *tissue* sensitivities (hypersensitivities), by far the most accurate and least expensive way to determine which foods are affecting you is to run a precise elimination/provocation trial using your own bodymind as the laboratory. The good news is, by conducting this dietary trial (which is safe, costs nothing but time and effort, and requires no prescription), you can expect to feel significantly better within a very short period of time.

Conducting a Successful Trial

Before beginning, it is absolutely *essential* you gain enough knowledge and a thorough understanding of all the *how's* and *why's* of success, so you will be able to do the elimination/provocation dietary trial 100% correctly. Read this chapter several times, as well as Chapters 7, 9 and 26 before embarking on this journey. In addition, I highly recommend keeping a detailed journal of everything you eat and drink, jotting down any symptoms or improvements you notice along the way. You may be reacting to many different foods, and combinations of foods, so it generally takes some careful detective work to sort through it all. And finally, I highly recommend lining up a support system, whether that be a spouse, partner or friend. Even better, find someone willing to conduct the trial along with you!

In the United States, the two most common culprits of hidden hypersensitivity symptoms caused by leaking peptides are *gluten* (such as wheat, rye, barley and cross-contaminated oats) and *casein* (milk and dairy). For this reason, begin by eliminating *at least* these two proteins. The next most common culprits are peanuts, tree nuts, eggs, fish, shellfish, corn and soybeans.[1] *Any* food can cause a hypersensitivity reaction, so pay attention to any suspicions you may have. Generally, the foods you eat frequently and/or crave the most should be at the top of your list of suspected offenders. For example, in China far more people have allergies to rice than wheat or dairy, because rice is a staple there.*

The human immune system will react to even the most *minute* traces of an offending protein, which is why anything less than 100% dietary elimination is a complete waste of time and energy. Simply "cutting down" on the troublesome foods will not work! If, for example, you suspect that the proteins in dairy (casein, whey and several others) are adversely affecting you, just giving up milk and cheese while continuing to eat yogurt would be a wasted trial. A correct dietary trial would involve complete elimination of *any and all* foods that contain traces of dairy proteins, and that includes its many different disguises.[2] Read all the ingredients! If any traces of the offending protein are accidentally ingested during the elimination period, the trial should be considered invalid and will need to be repeated from scratch.

Phase 1: Identify the Culprits

There are two ways to approach the elimination/provocation diet. The first is to eliminate the entire list of common and suspected reactive foods (wheat, dairy, peanuts, tree nuts, eggs, corn, fish, shellfish, soybeans and anything else you suspect) for two weeks, then begin the provocation phase one food at a time. The second is to conduct an elimination and provocation of only one food at a time (which takes longer but tends to be more accurate). After reading this chapter, choose the method that most suits your needs and personality.

---

* There is no need to despair over calcium deficiency from eliminating dairy. Contrary to the fictitious propaganda of the dairy industry, dairy products are a terrible form of calcium for human beings (I say this despite growing up on a dairy farm). The best sources of dietary calcium for humans are foods that are high in calcium *and* low in phosphorus, such as green leafy vegetables and, for infants, human breast milk. Cow's milk is the opposite, with a high phosphorus to calcium ratio. If your calcium needs cannot be met by diet alone, I highly recommend taking calcium hydroxyapatite with boron, the *only* form of calcium supplement proven to slow, halt or even reverse bone loss.[3]

With the first approach, you would eliminate all the foods listed in the previous paragraph for two weeks, which would potentially leave you with a diet of gluten-free grains (brown rice, wild rice, buckwheat, millet, quinoa, corn, sorghum, amaranth and montina)[4] plus green vegetables, fresh fruits, beans, potatoes and lean meats. At the end of the two weeks, choose *one* food protein to reintroduce in a small amount (for example, milk), noting any reactions or return of symptoms. This is the provocation phase in which you will "test" the eliminated food by eating a small amount of it to see if any reaction or symptoms occur. Trust me, your bodymind will let you know, loud and clear, whether or not it wants you to continue eating that particular food. If no reaction is noticed, continue eating your core group of foods along with the newly added food for another two weeks and then reintroduce a second food protein. However, if a reaction *was* noticed, stop eating that food. Go back to your core list, wait two more weeks to clear it out of your system, and then test another. And so forth.

The second approach involves testing each suspected food protein individually (or perhaps two at a time). For example, during the first two weeks, eliminate all traces of gluten. Then, do the provocation and note any symptoms. During the next two weeks, eliminate all traces of casein (continuing to stay *off* gluten if any reaction was noted at reintroduction). Continue on in this fashion until all suspected foods have been tested. Testing this way will take longer, but I believe it is less overwhelming for most people and in fact, more accurate. The only problem with this approach is, if you are reacting to a combination of two or more different food proteins, eliminating one while eating various others may give confusing results.

Remember, no matter which approach you choose, you must eliminate *all traces* of the suspected protein(s) from your diet for two full weeks, noticing how you feel. If your bothersome symptoms clear up during the elimination, only to return at provocation, congratulations! You have identified a food protein that has been adversely affecting your health. If you feel the same as you did before the elimination, either you don't have food sensitivities *or* there is another food (or foods) you are still eating that are wreaking havoc, such as refined carbohydrates. Continue this process, using your chosen approach, until you believe you have identified all the culprits. Next, it is time for phase two.

Phase 2: Reset the Immune System

The next phase of this process is complete elimination of your entire list of offending proteins for a six-month period. As explained in Chapters 9 and 26, it takes about six months for your immune system to "forget" its sensitivity, and in so doing, the addiction pattern is also broken. You can only reach that point if there is zero ingestion of any and all traces from start to finish. *Any cheating or accidental ingestion during the six-month period will only serve to keep the immune system exquisitely sensitive to the offending proteins indefinitely!*

It is important to understand that even though elimination of your offending food proteins can bring tremendous relief of symptoms, this alone cannot be considered a "cure." Until you deal with *why* you have food hypersensitivities, any dietary elimination approach will only meet with temporary success. If you have read this entire book, and are able to see the big picture of how everything ties together to create either disease or Wellness, you will understand why the only lasting approach to reversing food sensitivities is one that combines eliminating the offending substances, *while at the same time* reversing and healing leaky gut syndrome (LGS) by discharging the accumulated stored stress-effect burden in the hypothalamus. Keep in mind many patients with allergies also have Candida-related syndrome (C-RS) as a major contributor to their LGS and so will need to take action toward eradicating this parasite as well.

Glass House or Greener Pastures?

It would be nice if we could just eliminate one or two foods and move on with our lives. Unfortunately, if dietary elimination is the *only* approach taken, it often leads to a progressive narrowing of your available options. For example, if you start avoiding all foods containing casein and gluten, you will begin substituting other foods to take their place (rice, beans, corn, soy, etc.). Since the risk of immune system reaction tends to be proportional to the amount of exposure, there is a high risk of developing *new* hypersensitivities to the remaining foods you are now eating much more often, forcing you to start eliminating some of *these* as well. You may also find yourself reacting to various environmental triggers such as scented candles, perfume and so forth. As time goes on, you may find yourself living in a glass house, breathing filtered air and eating roasted platypus!

Approaching food hypersensitivities from a holistic perspective offers the advantage of beginning to experience a wider and wider exposure to life, as opposed to the inevitable progressive narrowing if the first approach (eliminating the offenders) is all that is done. The ideal approach is to combine dietary elimination with the 3LS of Wellness as described in Section IV of this book.

CHAPTER 28

Intracellular Magnesium

The freethinking of one age is the common sense of the next.

~ Matthew Arnold
(English poet and cultural critic, 1822–1888)

Magnesium: A Vital Macro-Mineral

Minerals are key to your good health. Your bodymind needs both micro-minerals (also known as "trace" minerals) and macro-minerals. The prefix "micro" refers to small or minute amounts, and the prefix "macro" refers to larger or more significant amounts. Trace minerals, as the name suggests, are only needed in trace amounts to catalyze most of the reactions the bodymind performs for optimal function. Once considered an unimportant *micro*-mineral, magnesium is now seen as *so* important to health that it has been reclassified as a macro-mineral. Examples of other common macro-minerals include calcium, iron, phosphorus and zinc.

Magnesium happens to be one of the most crucial minerals lost in the food refining process, causing as many as 80% of Americans to become deficient.[1] The refining process (which began in the 1890s) combined with increasingly deficient soils has created a situation in which over 75% of the foods we eat today no longer contain magnesium. Further adding to the problem, the increase in chemicals, environmental pollutants and toxic metals block our ability to metabolize and absorb this vital nutrient. The conventional medical paradigm is only now just beginning to recognize that not only does magnesium belong in the macro-mineral class, but that it may well be the most *important* neglected mineral of all.

The Many Cries of Deficiency

Magnesium deficiency has been shown to be a major cause of many common health complaints.[2] Common symptoms and chronic conditions indicative of magnesium deficiency include muscle tension ("bracing"), fatigue, insomnia, asthma, allergies, migraine headaches, many forms of hypoglycemia, brain chemistry disorders (including depression, anxiety, panic, mood swings, memory difficulties, etc.), PMS, osteoporosis, hypertension, cardiac dysrhythmia, congestive heart failure, fibromyalgia, muscle cramps or twitching, restless legs syndrome (RLS), seizures, stroke and more. Adequate magnesium levels are especially critical for pregnant women, patients with myocardial infarction and/or diabetes (a condition that depletes magnesium).[3]

Generally speaking, new concepts such as this usually take a full generation to begin to be accepted, and then another generation to be put into use by the profession. Pre-eclampsia during pregnancy is a classic example of the harm that can come from the overall lack of attention and seriousness with which conventional medicine views magnesium deficiency. Pre-eclampsia in an expectant mother is a cry for magnesium. Undetected, it can progress to full-blown toxemia—an emergency situation that is, despite all lack of a preventive approach, treated by immediately giving the mother one or more painful intramuscular injections of 50cc of magnesium sulfate.

If our medical system was set up to be more proactive about nutrition and prevention, all expectant mothers would be put on high doses of an easily absorbed form of magnesium throughout pregnancy and such emergencies would long be a thing of the past. As it is now, conventional doctors do not even give magnesium to women with a *history* of this condition in previous pregnancies, even though it is known that one episode almost guarantees the next! Given the facts, the refusal to acknowledge and utilize this simple preventive measure is, in my opinion, inexcusable.

Testing: Intracellular Versus Serum

Even though about 80% of the people in our country are deficient in magnesium, most conventional physicians fail to test for it. Of those who do, most are still ordering the worthless "serum magnesium" tests, which tell us nothing about the functional magnesium levels in the body. Magnesium is an *intracellular* mineral, therefore only the white or red blood cell "intracellular magnesium test" has any validity.[4]

Whether or not you choose to undergo formal testing for magnesium deficiency, the very best laboratory is the one nature gave you—the bodymind. Even if your intracellular magnesium test comes back within the "normal" range, your magnesium level may still be too low for *you*. If your bodymind suggests this is the case, a trial of a highly absorbable form of magnesium would easily determine whether supplementation would be beneficial for you.

Supplemental Magnesium: Oral Forms

Despite being one of the most important nutrients to the body, even high quality magnesium is among the most difficult minerals for the GI tract to absorb, especially when digestive efficiency begins to wane due to leaky gut syndrome (LGS). Magnesium oxide, the cheapest form of magnesium and the one most often found for sale, is practically worthless except as a laxative because it is absorbed so poorly. In my opinion, it is unethical to sell magnesium oxide as a nutritional supplement. The best supplemental forms of elemental magnesium are glycinate, ororate and aspartate. Of these three oral forms, glycinate is the most easily absorbed.

An unfortunate quirk about magnesium metabolism is that often, once levels are low enough to cause symptoms in a particular individual, the body may have already lost the ability to efficiently absorb magnesium through even the best oral supplementation. To find out whether this is the case for you, I recommend beginning with a therapeutic trial of two grams (2000 mg) of elemental magnesium glycinate, ororate or aspartate in a chelated oral supplement, twice per day (total 4 grams). Taking digestive enzymes and 200 mg vitamin B6 (a co-factor for magnesium) with each dose will enhance absorption.

High doses of magnesium and vitamin B6 are nontoxic, meaning it is almost impossible to be harmed by taking too much. If you experience intestinal upset or loose stools (with *any* form of magnesium), it is a sure sign that it is not being absorbed. If this occurs, or if no improvements are noticed after a few months on this trial, don't throw the baby out with the bathwater. It simply means that you will need to look into alternative magnesium options for a period of time.

Intravenous and Transdermal Magnesium

Anyone deficient enough in magnesium to have lost the ability to absorb it through oral supplementation will likely need a therapeutic trial of either intravenous (IV) infusions or a high quality topical magnesium product (absorbed through the skin, also called "transdermal"). The first option involves receiving at least two grams of elemental magnesium chloride (the most preferred form for intravenous use) via IV infusion three times a week for two weeks. These IV infusions can be injected virtually painlessly in about five minutes, without risks or negative side effects. The second option is to obtain a high-quality topical magnesium for transdermal absorption and use it as directed for at least one month.[5] By the end of the therapeutic trial period for the IV or topical magnesium, your bodymind will have made it clear whether or not you needed this (that is, did your symptoms improve?).

Whether you choose IV infusions or topical magnesium, continue taking *half* the dose of your oral magnesium supplementation, along with the described co-factors, at the same time. With your intracellular magnesium levels restored, you should now be able to take, *and absorb*, a much smaller maintenance dose of oral magnesium from that point on. To determine your maintenance dose, take at least one gram of elemental magnesium (glycinate, ororate or aspartate) twice a day for the first month. Then try cutting that dose in half. Although the average 150-pound person will maintain benefits with just 500 mg per day, dosage is very individual and is a matter of trial and error. If only you will listen, your bodymind will determine the correct maintenance dose for you.

CHAPTER 29

Essential Fatty Acids

If you cannot solve your problem, then what is the need of worrying? If you cannot solve it, then what is the need of worrying?

~ Shantideva
(8th-century Indian Buddhist scholar)

Why EFAs Are "Essential"

Several chapters throughout this book have recommended essential fatty acid (EFA) supplementation for individuals with certain chronic health conditions. As the term "essential fatty acids" implies, these nutrients are *essential* to the healthy function of many areas of metabolism.[1] Signs and symptoms of EFA deficiency include digestive problems and constipation; dry hair, skin and mucous membranes (such as chapped lips); fatigue and low endurance; arthritic disorders; poor immunity, allergies and chronic rashes; acne and sebaceous cysts; hormonal imbalance; depression and forgetfulness; high blood lipids (cholesterol, etc.), hypertension and cardiovascular disease.

A defining characteristic of all "vitamins" is that they cannot be made within the body and so *must* be obtained from outside sources (your diet). Similarly, EFAs cannot be made within the body and so could be thought of as "fat vitamins." (Likewise, essential amino acids could be thought of as "protein vitamins.") If your diet is not providing EFAs in adequate amounts, supplementation is highly recommended. This chapter gives instructions on how to perform a therapeutic trial so you can experience the benefits for yourself.

Individual EFA requirements vary greatly. The two basic types of EFAs we hear about most often are omega 3 and omega 6 fatty acids (omega 9 fatty acids are also essential, however the standard American diet provides more than enough of these). Although much depends on your dietary habits, most people are far more deficient in omega 3 than omega 6. Supplementing omega 6 *may* be unnecessary if your diet includes a fair amount of nuts, seeds and their oils.

Before purchasing EFAs, do some research to discover which manufacturers are the most reputable. Look for carefully prepared, high quality oils from the best sources available.[2] The best manufacturers pack their capsules in nitrogen or vacuum seal them, so they will not need refrigeration *until* the bottle has been opened. Once opened, refrigeration is extremely important because oxygen perfuses through the capsule walls and can lead to rancidity. Since consuming *any* rancid oils (including nuts, seeds and cooking oils) is counterproductive to health, be sure to store *all* oils, and foods containing oil, in the fridge or freezer after opening.

Therapeutic Trial: Omega 3 and 6

To discover how EFA supplementation might benefit your health, I find that the quickest results are obtained by starting a dose that is high enough to benefit nearly everyone, then slowly reducing that dose in scheduled increments until your bodymind lets you know the lowest effective dose for *you*. There is no danger, except to your pocketbook, in taking more EFAs than your body needs.

EFAs are always best taken in *at least* two divided doses throughout the day. If you weigh over 150 pounds, begin by taking approximately 5000 mg omega 3 and 1500 mg omega 6 daily. If you weigh less than 150 pounds, begin by taking or approximately 3670 mg omega 3 and 1100 mg omega 6 daily. Again, use these suggestions as a guideline, keeping in mind that many people will not even *need* the omega 6.

The recommended dosages refer to the *active ingredients* in each serving. Be sure to look carefully at the fine print on the back of the bottle to find out how much active ingredient is in each capsule or spoonful, and be prepared to do some math. For example, for a bottle that states on the front label *omega 3 fish oil concentrate, 1000 mg capsules*, the back label will likely reveal there are only about 300 mg of the active ingredients per capsule. Therefore, a large number of capsules will have to be taken in order to get the correct amount of active ingredients for the trial period. For those who cannot swallow the (fairly large) capsules, liquid EFAs are usually available in the refrigerated section of your local health food store.

The active ingredients in omega 3 fatty acids are eicosapentaenoic acid (EPA) and docosahexaenoic acid (DHA). The active ingredients in omega 6 oils are gamma linolenic acid (GLA), alpha linolenic acid (ALA) and linolenic acid (LA). Due to the obvious limitation of working with capsules containing various amounts of active ingredient each, dosages will likely need to be rounded up or down to the nearest desired amount. For example, if your goal is 1250 mg of omega 3 and the back label shows each capsule contains 300 mg of the active ingredient, taking four capsules would be your closest bet (1200 mg).

Breakdown of EFAs

Omega 3 Fatty Acid Sources

cold water fish oils (least expensive)

flaxseed oil (slightly more expensive)

Omega 3 Active Ingredients

DHA (docosahexaenoic acid)

EPA (eicosapentaenoic acid)

Omega 6 Fatty Acid Sources

borage oil (least expensive)

black currant oil (mid-priced)

evening primrose oil (most expensive)

Omega 6 Active Ingredients

GLA (gamma linolenic acid)

LA (linoleic acid)

Determining Maintenance Dose

Although many people notice health improvements within the first few days of high-dose supplementation, it actually takes a few months of consistent dosing to get the full effect. Once benefits are clearly realized, determine your maintenance dose by cutting the original dose in half. Notice whether your good results are maintained over the next few months. If so, repeat this process by cutting the dose in half again. Continue decreasing the dose every few months, paying close attention to your bodymind, because eventually you will notice some of your symptoms beginning to return. This temporary discomfort is just part of the process of helping you determine your lowest effective dose. When symptoms begin to reappear, it simply means your *most recent* dose cut was one too many for your individual EFA requirements. At that point, simply return to your previous lowest effective dose and remain on it indefinitely for maintenance.

As an example, let's say you begin your trial by taking 5000 mg omega 3 and 1500 mg omega 6 fatty acids (in divided doses, twice a day). Soon, you notice significant improvements in your arthritis pain and stiffness. Your skin feels less dry and your acne seems to be clearing up. Even your depression seems to be lifting. After 60 days of improvements, you cut the dose in half (2500 mg omega 3 and 750 mg omega 6), continuing this dose for two more months. You are pleased to find you still feel great, with no return of your previous symptoms. You then cut the dose in half again (1250 mg omega 3 and 375 mg omega 6). Two more months pass at this dose, and your benefits are still maintained. You cut the dose in half yet again (625 mg omega 3 and 180 mg omega 6). This time, within a few weeks you notice your old symptoms returning. Your bodymind is telling you that your most recent EFA dose fell just below your individual requirements. You then go back to your previous *effective* dose (1250 mg omega 3 and 375 mg omega 6), and maintain that dose indefinitely.

As mentioned previously, you could continue taking the highest dose forever without hurting anything but your wallet. Cost is the only reason for experimenting to discover your personal lowest effective dose. If taking EFAs significantly improves any outward symptoms that have been troubling you, it is a sure sign your entire system has been needing them for many other metabolic pathways as well. Therefore, you'll be pleasantly surprised to begin noticing additional unexpected improvements in your health. This is just another example of the multiple benefits of holistic therapies.

CHAPTER 30

Avoiding Unnecessary Antibiotics

The desire to take medicine is perhaps the greatest feature which distinguishes man from animals.

~ Sir William Osler
(Canadian physician, historian and author, 1849–1919)

Infections: Bacterial or Viral?

Make no mistake about it, countless lives have been saved by the proper and timely administration of antibiotic medications. Beginning with Sir Alexander Fleming's groundbreaking discovery of penicillin in 1926, several different classes of antibiotics have been developed to combat numerous potentially life-threatening bacterial infections. The discovery and proper use of antibiotics is just one historical example of the many areas in which conventional medicine shines.

Antibiotics were originally designed to be used only after an infected area has been cultured and laboratory analysis has demonstrated a susceptible bacterium. *Only* if a bacterial infection has been identified at the lab, *and* the specific antibiotic sensitivity is determined, should the correct (let alone *any*) antibiotic then be prescribed. Specific conditions caused by very specific bacteria can only be helped by taking very specific antibiotics. Unfortunately, with the exception of the commonly performed strep throat culture, many physicians are in the sloppy habit of skipping culture and lab analysis altogether.

Antibiotics work *only* for bacterial infections and even then, *only* if the particular bacteria strain is susceptible to the particular antibiotic prescribed. There is *no such thing* as an antibiotic for viral infections. Every doctor knows this simple fact, however, too many patients do not. Some people (especially parents of young children) become almost frantic about obtaining antibiotics at the first sign of every cold or flu, believing the medication will somehow make the illness go away faster or prevent it from "turning into something worse." With colds or the flu, neither scenario is remotely possible!

The most common conditions for which antibiotics are prescribed are ear, sinus and throat infections. However, research has shown the majority of these types of infection are *viral* or allergic in nature. Of the remaining minority that are *bacterial*, nearly all would clear up on their own if given a little time and the standard supportive techniques, such as rest, fluids and proper nutrition. Since many doctors are either not willing to argue with (and risk losing) their patients, antibiotics are frequently prescribed upon patient request. When the patient feels better a few days later, they mistakenly credit the antibiotics and their doctor instead of realizing that any improvement gained is due to a combination of the placebo effect and nature running its course (despite the *interference* of the antibiotic).

The Placebo Effect

A controlled, double-blind study is one in which about half the participants are given a real treatment and the other half are given a placebo (a fake treatment such as a sugar pill). Neither the study participants nor the researchers know who is being given what. The purpose of such studies is to determine whether positive effects noted are due to treatment itself or to belief in the treatment—the power of suggestion and belief. Actually, the placebo effect is a wonderful thing. It is proof of the powerful bodymind connection, demonstrating how positive thoughts and beliefs can literally heal the body.

In medical school, we were taught that the average positive placebo effect in any controlled double-blind study was about 30%. Within the last few decades, we've discovered that the actual, real-life positive placebo effect is much higher. We also were taught that when you combine a doctor who believes in the effectiveness of the medication being prescribed with a patient who knows what that medication is, and has faith in the doctor, the positive placebo effect rises to an amazing

70%! Naturally, young children are even more susceptible to the placebo effect than most adults because they are very suggestible and have such a high degree of belief in what the trusted adults in their lives tell them.

As explained in Chapter 10, you can expect to be over the symptoms of the common cold virus within about two weeks, and the flu within about three weeks. The one symptom most likely to persist beyond these time frames is cough. Patients who understand these facts are more likely to allow a viral illness to "run its course" instead of rushing into the doctor's office demanding treatment. On occasion, the original virus can spawn a bacterial infection that *might* require antibiotic treatment. Therefore, it is good to know when a visit to the doctor might be warranted.

Secondary Bacterial Infections

Any time an illness onsets from a viral or bacterial infection in the body, fever is normal and to be expected. Fever is the body's natural way of fighting off the illness. In fact, I never recommend trying to reduce a fever until or unless it has risen above 102 degrees. As just stated, there are occasions when fever is a sign that what began as a viral infection (such as cold or flu) may have led to a *secondary* bacterial infection. You can be suspicious of this if either of the following two scenarios occur: symptoms that were progressively getting better suddenly worsen again and/or a fever reappears several days after the original fever has gone.

Even when your symptoms seem to be lingering for weeks on end (as cough most commonly does), if there is no fever, there is likely *no* secondary bacterial infection requiring antibiotic treatment. In most cases, lingering symptoms can be attributed to allergies and/or hypersensitivities perpetuating the illness through inflammation of the sinus or bronchial passages. This is often the case even if you think you don't have "allergies." People can even be allergic to the cold virus itself, which is the reason many cold remedies contain an antihistamine ingredient.

If your illness displays the warning signs just described, the only way to know for sure whether you have a secondary bacterial infection is to get a culture for pathogenic bacteria, known as a "culture and sensitivity" test. Unfortunately, very few docs do cultures other than for Strep anymore, and it would probably take an act of Congress to stop this sloppy practice. Since it is *impossible* to know whether a bacterial infection is present without sending a culture to the lab, and since each bacterial strain has a different antibiotic sensitivity, I recommend you *insist* on getting a culture.

Doctors in the United States, who know the facts full well, are still prescribing antibiotics for cold symptoms about 60% of the time, at a cost of $37.5 million per year.[1] Any doctor who prescribes antibiotics without first performing a culture and sensitivity test is making assumptions and taking the easy way out by sending you off with a prescription "just in case." If the only harm of this practice was a little money down the drain, perhaps the unnecessary use of antibiotics wouldn't be such a big deal. Unfortunately, a *much* higher price is being paid, both individually and collectively.

Treating It *Just in Case?*

The human body comes equipped with its own disease-fighting mechanism—the highly capable immune system. When allowed to do its job without unnecessary interference, the immune system develops its own natural antibodies against infection, making the immune system stronger.

Improper use of antibiotics actually hinders your natural ability to recover, damaging the immune system *and* your long-term health. And if that weren't enough, every individual who takes unnecessary antibiotics, even once, puts the entire human species at risk by adding to the increasing antibiotic-resistant strains of bacteria within the population. What will we do when the newest "super-bug" emerges and we have *no* antibiotic that can touch it?

The four most common scenarios that are putting the entire human population at risk for resistant strains of bacteria are: taking antibiotics when not necessary (such as for viral infections or low-risk, self-limiting bacterial infections), taking the wrong antibiotic for a particular strain of infection, taking "broad-spectrum" antibiotics when not absolutely necessary, and/or failing to take a properly prescribed antibiotic as directed for the full course of treatment. Perhaps the most dangerous practice of all is indiscriminately feeding antibiotics to livestock in doses inadequate for curing anything but perfect for developing resistant strains of bacteria.[2]

If only they were used properly, we would not be in the antibiotic-resistance crisis we are in today. As more and more of our antibiotic drugs have become increasingly useless, pharmaceutical companies have followed suit by developing broad-spectrum antibiotics designed to kill the widest possible variety of bacteria. Instead of saving these "big guns" for the truly life-threatening conditions, doctors have been prescribing them for just about anything, including colds, flu, simple ear infections, chronic acne and prophylactic use of antibiotics in dental procedures for patients with heart valve lesions.[3] This is known as the "shotgun" approach.

Broad-spectrum antibiotics effectively kill off the normal flora population present in the healthy gut ecology (the "good" bacteria), resulting in dysbiosis. In fact, broad-spectrum antibiotics are often far more effective at destroying healthy flora than they could ever be at selectively attacking any possible disease-causing bacteria that might be present.

As explained in Section II of this book, both leaky gut syndrome (LGS) and Candida-related syndrome (C-RS) also lead to dysbiosis. All of these conditions serve as precursors to so many other increasingly common illnesses of our modern times, many of which are not currently recognized by conventional physicians. In a now vicious cycle, sparked by the unnecessary use of antibiotics, LGS and C-RS further depress your immune system. The more depressed your immunity, the more susceptible you will be to new and more frequent infections of the ears, nose, throat, skin, etc. in the long run. Just consider the "new disease of the month" phenomenon happening before our very eyes!

It can be difficult to accept truths that go against our cherished illusions, but ignorance is rarely bliss. Now that you understand the facts about the risks of unnecessary antibiotics, spread the word. As I always say, an enlightened and aware public is its own best protection!

CHAPTER 31

Hot Compresses

An ounce of prevention is worth a pound of cure.

~ Henry de Bracton
(English jurist and law writer, 1210–1268)

A First Course of Action

Moist, hot compresses are an extremely effective means of combating localized infections of the skin. A truism of the body is as follows: Any space that is supposed to drain but cannot will always get infected, *and* vice versa, any space that drains normally will never get, or stay, infected. When it comes to skin infections, fluids underneath the skin are unable to drain. Acute skin infections present as pain, redness and inflammation. The conventional method of dealing with such infections is to lance, drain, then prescribe antibiotics. These expensive and painful trips to the doctor can almost always be prevented by using moist, hot compresses as your first course of action.

Some of the most common types of skin infections are caused by the accumulation of sebum in the pocket of a cyst (such as acne, sebaceous or pilonidal cysts). Other very common types of skin infections include boils, carbuncles, ingrown hairs, ingrown toenails, impetigo and bug bites, as well as infected cuts, burns and puncture wounds. If you want to familiarize yourself with various types of skin infections for the purpose of self-diagnosis, I recommend consulting any good full-color dermatology atlas at your local library.

Without risk, pain or expense, hot compresses eliminate skin infections faster and more reliably than any antibiotic. They not only promote the necessary drainage that naturally resolves such infections, they also increase circulation, bringing your body's own immune cells and antibodies to the area. The only contraindication to the use of hot compresses would be for diabetics, who should never apply heat below the knees without professional oversight.

Moist heat works better than dry heat because the moisture helps keep sticky fluids from drying and blocking the opening through which the infection needs to drain. Along this same line, anything with a great deal of fluid to drain (like a boil) will drain better between hot compress applications if you keep some type of oily substance like plain white petroleum jelly over the opening.

Application Instructions

For acute inflammation, apply moist hot compresses for five minutes every hour according to the following instructions. Fold or roll a washcloth into the smallest surface area possible. Dip that portion of the cloth into hot water from your tap and apply directly to the site of the infection. Add more hot water to the cloth as necessary to keep it hot enough to be slightly uncomfortable for the full five minutes. Never use boiling or scalding hot water! It is neither necessary nor desirable to risk a burn by making the water too hot.

The goal is to create a compress that can be applied to *just* the infected area without applying it to a significant amount of the surrounding normal skin. Many people have been mistakenly taught to *soak* in hot water for skin infections, such as taking a sitz bath for a pilonidal cyst. Soaking a large area is not the best solution because it eliminates the most important factor involved in how the heat works: the *ratio* of the area being heated to the rest of the body. Hot compresses work by concentrating circulation from your entire body into the precise area where it is needed. In general, the more locally you apply the heat, the more this ratio is maximized and the more effective the result.

Once improvement is noticed (a reduction in pain, redness and swelling), you can decrease the frequency from hourly to once every 2–3 hours and continue until the area is normal. If, after following the above instructions exactly, you do not experience improvement within twenty-four hours (much faster than any antibiotic could work), consult your doctor.

CHAPTER 32

Gentle Rebounding

The superior man is modest in his speech,
but exceeds in his actions.

~ Confucius
(Chinese philosopher, 551 BC–479 BC)

Bouncing for Health

Rebounding is a simple, enjoyable and non-strenuous activity that almost anyone can do to improve many aspects of general health. Rebounding improves lymphatic circulation and drainage, assists with body detoxification, enhances muscle tone, strengthens the immune system, improves breathing capacity, and so much more. Rebounding involves bouncing on a mini-trampoline (also known as a rebounder) or bouncing while sitting on a large inflatable exercise ball. Although these items *can* be used for more vigorous activity such as Aerobic Exercise, only very gentle bouncing is necessary for the purposes described in this chapter.

There are many different types and brands of rebounders available on the market today. The main differences are price and the quality of the springs, mat and frame. If you weigh less than 200 pounds, or if you just want to commit to a short trial of this activity, an inexpensive rebounder will probably suffice. If you weigh over 200 pounds or plan on using it more extensively, consider purchasing a more durable rebounder.

The health benefits of gentle rebounding have very little to do with this being "exercise," since it isn't even necessary for your feet to lift off the surface of the mat (or your buttocks off the surface of the ball) when bouncing. Most of the benefits accrue from the effects of the reciprocal up and down motion itself. This motion, as I will explain, facilitates the release of toxins from various body tissues and speeds up their transport, via the lymph system, to locations where they can exit the body.[1]

How Rebounding Detoxifies the Body

In nature, matter exists in three forms: crystalline (solid), amorphous (liquid) and vapor (gas). A good example of this is water. Ice is crystalline, water is amorphous and steam is vapor. Most human body tissues exist in the amorphous form. Toxins *also* tend to be bound and stored in the amorphous form within the fat and protein makeup of the body.

Most bodily protein is within the organs and structural aspects, such as muscles, ligaments, tendons and fascia. It was previously believed that proteins on this planet (one gravity, 1-G) were always amorphous. Then about thirty years ago, it was discovered that proteins actually become more thoroughly amorphous at two gravities (2-G) and tend to crystallize at zero gravities (0-G). Why is this important? Just as water tends to purify itself during crystallization, so too, toxins tied up in amorphous protein tend to be released when the molecule becomes crystalline.

The up and down motion of rebounding converts the body's proteins from 2-G (the bottom of the bounce) to 0-G (the top of the bounce)—back and forth from amorphous to crystalline with each bounce. The up and down motion of rebounding also dramatically facilitates more efficient lymphoid circulation. Each conversion causes the molecules to release more of the bound toxins into the blood and thereby to the liver—the major detoxification organ of the bodymind. Whatever the liver cannot detoxify is excreted via the bile into the gut or leaked back into the blood, neither of which is desirable. Given this knowledge, it becomes clear why holistic practitioners focus on the importance of boosting detoxification pathways in and to the liver.[2]

A note about the liver: The liver is the organ most capable of regenerating itself after damage—especially if the problem is caught *before* the cells are dead. You can help protect your liver by avoiding things known to damage it, such as alcohol, environmental chemicals and certain medications such as acetaminophen (read your package insert). Many holistic liver cleansing methods such as castor oil packs (made famous by Edgar Cayce), coffee enemas and liver-gallbladder cleanses available on the market.[3] Supplements shown to be supportive include alpha-lipoic acid and milk thistle, both of which are safe and will not interfere with any conventional treatments.

Although most toxins go directly to the liver via the blood, the lymphatic system drains some of the toxins to the cisterna chyli (a large pocket in the lower chest/upper abdomen), which empties into the right atrium of the heart. The heart then pumps this blood to the skin, lungs and kidneys for excretion. Therefore, within the first two days, expect to experience signs of your body releasing toxins (such as increased perspiration, body odor and bad breath). These unpleasant signs will pass in time and can be viewed as positive evidence of the effectiveness of rebounding for detoxification.

Benefits will be achieved with only ten minutes of gentle rebounding, twice a day. Although additional time is better, rebounding more than six times per day will likely bring diminishing returns. As with all the holistic approaches recommended throughout this book, I recommend making a list of all your chronic symptoms before beginning, then keeping a journal for the next several months to track your progress.

Rebounding and Emphysema

Back in the late '70s or early '80s, I read an article about rebounding and emphysema published by the physical therapy department at the University of Michigan Medical School. The article reported that the mild up and down motion from very gentle bounding on a mini-trampoline significantly improved both the functional breathing capacity and the pulmonary function of patients with severe emphysema, a pathological accumulation of air in the lung tissues that makes it difficult to exhale.

The improvement in emphysema was *separate from* the exercise aspect of rebounding, since someone else could do the bouncing while the patient simply sat in the middle of the trampoline. At the time, I was still naive about the pervasive efforts of my profession at suppressing this type of information. I neglected to save the article, falsely assuming the findings would be expanded upon and eventually become the "standard of practice" in this country. Instead, this valuable discovery has been swept under the rug like so many other approaches that do not profit the allopathic monopoly. This is especially inexcusable, since conventional MDs have no effective solution for this miserable condition, and emphysema patients deserve to be informed of alternative options that can make a difference in their quality of life.

If you have emphysema, I recommend getting a rebounder for your home and bouncing on it, very gently, for about ten minutes twice a day. Even just sitting on the trampoline and rhythmically waving your forearms up and down will create the up and down motion needed to get results. If your disease is so advanced that you are unable to accomplish any of this by yourself, find a friend willing to bounce for you while you sit in the center of the mini-trampoline. That effort alone would be enough to bring noticeable results within a few short weeks. As your condition improves, you may be able to rebound more independently.

CHAPTER 33

Applied Kinesiology

Our own physical body possesses a wisdom which we who inhabit the body lack.

~ Henry Miller
(American novelist and painter, 1891–1980)

"Muscle Testing"

Applied kinesiology (AK) is a fun and interesting way to learn to pay attention to what your bodymind is trying to tell you. Also known as "muscle testing," AK was first developed in 1964 by American chiropractor George Goodheart. The science is based on the belief that within every person is an innate intelligence that not only heals us, but is also attempting to communicate with us. One of the most valuable aspects of AK is that it can assist you in discovering which foods, supplements and other substances (or even frequencies) are most compatible and beneficial—or conversely, least compatible and potentially harmful—for your unique bodymind system.

Most chiropractors are trained in this technique, and many use it with their clients on a regular basis. The only limits of AK are that it is best performed with a partner and it takes a fair amount of practice to learn how to perform it consistently and reliably. Not everyone will master the technique. People who are in touch with their intuition (something we are all born with) tend to have greater success.

The only real valuable thing is intuition.

~ Albert Einstein (1879–1955)

How to Perform AK

For the purposes of this book, the goal of using AK will be to help you determine the degree of positive or negative effect that various substances are having on your internal functions. Although it is possible to learn self-testing techniques, the description that follows will require a partner.

Begin by establishing a baseline. Have the person being tested hold one arm out to the side of the body, from the shoulder, level with the floor. The elbow must be kept straight. The tester will then apply a quick, firm (but not forceful) downward pressure at the wrist area and subjectively measure how "strong" the entire arm is (how much resistance there is to pushing the arm down). When this baseline test is done properly, the arm stays fairly firm and strong with only a slight bounce from the pressure. This is what is known as a "positive" response.

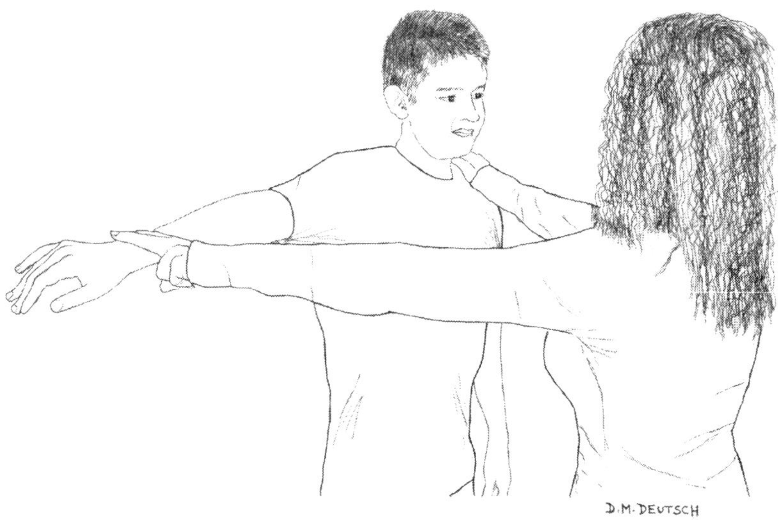

AK: "Muscle Testing"

Next, allow the arm to relax normally and choose a substance to test. I recommend beginning with sugar since it is a known negative stressor to the body and will therefore be the most reliable for demonstrating how

AK works. For accurate results, do not ingest any sugars or refined carbohydrates for two hours prior to testing. Place a small amount of sugar on the tongue then muscle test the arm again, in exactly the same way, being careful to use the same amount of pressure as before. Typically, the arm will go "weak," meaning the tester can now easily push the arm down (the person being tested can no longer hold the arm strongly and firmly in its original position). About 95% of people who muscle test sugar in this way lose between 30–98% of their strength within ten seconds of tasting the sugar. Even just one grain of sugar typically weakens the muscles for about fifteen minutes.

Everything Is Energy!

Once you have familiarized yourself with the procedure, you can experiment with testing other substances such as foods, supplements and medications. Do your best to remain in a neutral frame of mind, since strong expectations toward any specific result will often affect the accuracy of the testing. Keep in mind that when your muscle test shows a negative response to a substance (meaning it is energetically incompatible), every internal organ system—including the immune system—reduces its efficiency to the same degree that the tested muscle was weakened.

Given that everything in the universe consists of energetic vibrations, the most intuitive AK practitioners have discovered that similar information can often be obtained by simply holding the substance in the palm of your hand and then holding that hand over the solar plexus, noting any inner "yes" or inner "no."

A hand dynamometer is an inexpensive device that measures changes in muscle strength, and can therefore be used as a mechanical way of performing AK. Athletes use the more expensive versions to keep track of their progress in training various muscle groups. In my opinion, AK has certain advantages over such devices, but for the uninitiated beginner, skeptic or anyone who just wants to try testing a few simple substances, a dynamometer may be more reliable and believable.

For more information on Applied Kinesiology, I highly recommend reading *Your Body Doesn't Lie* by John Diamond, MD and *Energy Medicine* by Donna Eden (who uses and teaches AK to discover exactly which foods and supplements—including specific brands and dosages—are best for herself and her clients).[1] In addition, find a chiropractor in your local area who is trained in this technique and willing to work with you on perfecting it. With a little practice and persistence, you may find it's accuracy to be so impressive, you begin using muscle testing on a daily basis to receive feedback that will enhance all your efforts toward Wellness.

APPENDICES

Become an Active Participant
in Your Own Health Care

APPENDIX A

The Doctor-Patient Relationship

Two-Way Communication

Defined as the entry point into the conventional health-care system, your primary care physician makes the decisions that determine the accessibility, cost and quality of care you receive. He or she is in charge of ordering diagnostic tests, referring you to specialists and coordinating the efforts of everyone involved.

By the time you pick up the phone to call your doctor, you have already weighed a number of facts and decided that you need help. Once in the exam room, it is your job to communicate, in as clear a manner as possible, what the current problem is. If you withhold information (for example, due to embarrassment) or forget to include important details, decisions regarding your care may be off point. Once you have done your part, the doctor can follow suit, using his or her medical knowledge and experience to assist you in choosing the most appropriate approach to the problem. In other words, the doctor-patient relationship must be a *team effort*, not a dictatorship.

The "Doctor as God" Illusion

Over the past several generations, there has been a certain prevailing mystique surrounding doctors in our society known as the "Doctor as God" illusion. The (mostly subconscious) message behind this illusion is that we are blameless victims of disease, therefore our only hope is to get a doctor to fix or "save" us.

For some patients, once a doctor's diagnosis (educated guess) has tumbled forth from lips or pen, it is as if it is cast in stone. These people have been raised since birth to accept the treatment plan and prognosis as factual without question—in other words, agree with the diagnosis, have the surgery, take the pills and hope for the best. Furthermore, the diagnosis often becomes a personal label, added to the list of any other diseases and disorders with which they identify themselves. This misguided approach often strips patients of the self-responsibility needed to move *Beyond Disease Care*.

Despite the mystique, doctors are *not* all-knowing, infallible and beyond reproach. If you have been conditioned to believe that the doctor is always right and/or always knows best, think again. Keep in mind, the word "doctor" means "teacher." Any patient who disagrees with any aspect of the doctor's assessment and plan of action has the right (and the responsibility) to question it and/or seek a second opinion.

Think of doctors as consultants you are paying in order to use their training and experience as a tool for diagnosing, explaining and/or managing a health problem you feel you are incapable of handling yourself. In other words, the whole purpose of any doctor-patient encounter is to promote your best interests and ultimate well-being! *You* are the one who is doing all the suffering, paying all the fees and expending all the effort. You are also ultimately the one who will either reap all the benefits or suffer all the consequences of any mutually-agreed upon treatment decision.

As a physician, I'm going to let you in on a little secret. When it comes to chronic disease, diagnoses often arrive after a process of elimination (ruling out everything the condition is *not*). When no definitive cause can be found, doctors typically assign a general diagnostic label that actually goes nowhere in explaining the "why" behind your suffering. Even worse, I've known doctors who would practically defend their diagnoses to the death, lest their image and reputation be at risk. The best doctors are those who are willing to acknowledge and admit that despite doing their best, there may be errors in both diagnosis *and* proposed courses of action. You have the right to question your doctor, and your doctor has the right to be wrong.

Never put your doctor's ego above your health!

Patient Education and Compliance

Assuming the doctor's diagnosis is correct and the instructions given are safe and appropriate, patient education is by far the most powerful treatment that can be given. The unfortunate reality, however, is that tight schedules rarely allow time for this, and even with the instructions that *are* given, patient compliance is generally poor for many reasons. Patients may misunderstand or forget the doctor's instructions, or are simply too busy and disorganized to keep it all straight.

Exit interviews of patients leaving the doctor's office have shown that patients only remember about 30% of the instructions given. If interviewed the next day, these same patients can recall only about 10%. This is like going to the grocery store, shopping for an hour, standing in the checkout line, paying for your purchase, then throwing 70% of your items into the dumpster on your way out. Then, it's as if you open your refrigerator the next day only to find one-third of what you had left is still in there. Ultimately, it is up to *you* to decide the value of the information your doctor has given you.

A wise and intuitive doctor will make a shrewd evaluation of your personality before determining the best possible way to approach you. For some patients, an authoritarian approach is effective, but for others, it is the least productive. Some people would not dream of following a doctor's instructions without first gaining a thorough understanding of what is going on. Others are in denial of their illness and therefore cannot tolerate being involved in the management of their condition so will not listen to explanations.

Quality of Care

Just as the doctor will be making assessments about you, you have every right to make your own assessments about him or her. If you are the type of person who researches everything for yourself, you will want to find a doctor who doesn't operate from ego—one that will be open to your own research findings and admit that s/he doesn't always know more than you do. Indeed, the best doctor-patient relationships require a team effort. If you have multiple chronic symptoms, you will want a holistic doctor who is trained to look at the big picture instead of one who can't see the forest for the trees.

If you spend far more time in the waiting room than the exam room, and consistently go home feeling as though little or nothing was actually accomplished, it's time to change providers. The ideal providers view the doctor-patient relationship as a team effort, fully including you in the management of your own medical care, including being generally open and interested in hearing about (and learning from) any alternatives you have tried that worked for you.

What doctors do when treating patients is called "practice" for a reason. The bottom line is, nobody knows your body better than you do. Any doctor unwilling to listen to your gut feelings about your body is not one I would recommend keeping.

Choosing a Practitioner

Whether you prefer conventional or alternative practitioners, or a combination of both, your best protection is to be fully educated on *all* available options.[1] A great first step in that education is reading this book several times, conducting further research wherever indicated. The next step is implementing the 3LS of Wellness lifestyle changes described in Section IV of this book. The solutions are here. The only question is, are you ready to put forth the effort to be well?

Find a Holistic Practitioner

For assistance, contact any of the following:

- **American Holistic Medical Association (AHMA):** www.holisticmedicine.org. (216) 292-6644.
- **American Holistic Nursing Association (AHNA):** www.ahna.org. (800) 278-2462.
- **International Academy of Preventive Medicine (IAPM):** www.iapm.org. (800) 296-3651.
- **Bastyr University (Integrating Natural Health Arts and Sciences):** www.bastyr.edu. (425) 823-1300.

APPENDIX B

Symptoms Quick Reference

The following alphabetical list of common health complaints is provided as a reference to help you determine if your symptoms may warrant medical attention. Being educated with this information ahead of time will increase the effectiveness of your doctor-patient communication and the accuracy of your treatment plan.

Use the information only as a guide. Whether you have any of the warning signs listed or not, if you feel for any reason that you need medical attention, do not hesitate to contact your doctor or seek emergency attention!

Abdominal Pain

Abdominal pain can be one of the most difficult complaints to diagnose. Occasional heartburn or indigestion can be treated with antacids. However, if there is no relief within 30 minutes, or if there is *any* doubt that heartburn or indigestion is the cause of your discomfort, an office visit is indicated. Call your doctor if any of the following symptoms are present:

- Fever (one degree elevation or higher)
- Constant or severe pain
- Pain located in upper abdomen
- Pain located in lower right abdomen
- Additional pain with urination
- Vomiting blood
- Blood in a bowel movement
- Patient is under age 10

- Patient is pregnant
- Unusual vaginal discharge

Bumps, Bruises, Strains and Sprains

For any injury that produces swelling, apply ice or cold packs directly to the site of the swelling as much as tolerated for the first twenty-four hours, being sure to protect the skin with a towel. Call your doctor if any of the following symptoms are present:

- Severe swelling
- Severe pain
- Suspected fracture

Chest Pain

Continuous chest pain needs to be evaluated by a physician. If the pain comes and goes, or if it only hurts when you breathe, it is probably a non-emergency. If you think your pain may be coming from your heart, seek immediate medical attention. Call your doctor if any of the following symptoms are present:

- Constant or severe pain
- Pain associated with exertion
- Patient has a heart condition
- Patient has any chronic diseases
- Irregular pulse
- Nausea or vomiting

Cough

Coughing is a symptom, not an illness. Cough can be a symptom of anything from a cold to heart failure, so it is important to determine the cause. When a cough continues to persist after a viral infection such as cold or flu, the most likely cause is the act of coughing itself. (See Chapter 10.) Call your doctor if any of the following symptoms are present:

- Temperature above 100 degrees
- Pulse above 100 beats per minute
- Cough duration more than one week without cold or flu
- Chest pain
- Wheezing or shortness of breath
- Coughing up material
- Swelling anywhere, especially in ankles or face
- Patient smokes or has any chronic diseases

Lacerations

Any laceration (cut) to the skin must be immediately cleaned with antibacterial soap and water. Direct pressure over a cut will control bleeding in most cases. Once bleeding stops, leave the wound open to the air. If bleeding is excessive, keep pressure on the wound and call your doctor. If you can pull the skin apart, sutures or other methods of repair are needed.

Dizziness, Weakness or Blackouts

Dizziness (vertigo), weakness and/or blackouts can have many different causes. Often such symptoms accompany a self-limited illness such as cold or flu. Call your doctor if any of the following symptoms or circumstances are present:

- Fever (one degree elevation or higher)
- Abnormal pulse rate
- Recent head injury
- Difficulty speaking or swallowing
- Weakness or numbness only on one side
- Headache or chest pain
- Nausea, vomiting or diarrhea
- Patient taking medications
- Patient has any chronic diseases

Headache

Most acute headaches are due to nervous tension and can be safely treated at home with relaxation techniques and over-the-counter pain medications. (See Chapter 12.) Call your doctor if any of the following symptoms or circumstances are present:

- Fever (one degree elevation or higher)
- Severe pain
- Neck stiffness
- Recent blow to the head
- Any blackouts or loss of consciousness
- Visual changes (double vision, blurring)
- Difficulty speaking or changes in speech
- Patient has, or has ever had, high blood pressure
- Headache is "different" than previous headaches

Nausea, Vomiting and Diarrhea

Most vomiting and diarrhea can be attributed to a virus or food-borne illness and will therefore be self-limiting. The most important goal is to avoid dehydration. Sip only clear liquids (any liquid you can read newsprint through) and avoid irritating foods and drinks until symptoms have been gone for twenty-four hours. Call your doctor if any of the following symptoms or circumstances are present:

- Fever (one degree elevation or higher)
- Recent head injury
- Yellow discoloration of skin or eyes
- Blood in stool
- Vomiting any blood
- Constant or severe abdominal pain
- Pain in upper abdomen
- Significant dehydration

- Patient is diabetic
- Patient is taking Digitalis
- Symptoms do not improve for three or more days

Runny Nose, Hay Fever and Sinus Problems

These symptoms can be aggravating but in most cases are not serious. If the drainage comes about the same time every year, allergy is likely the cause. Call your doctor if any of the following symptoms are present:

- Temperature above 101 degrees
- Pulse above 100 beats per minute
- Pain in the face, forehead or behind the eyes
- Significant headache
- Neck stiffness
- Sore throat
- Yellow or green nasal discharge

Skin Rash

Skin rashes are common complaints. Many are due to allergy or contact with an irritant such as poison ivy, chemicals or harsh soaps. Symptoms can often be somewhat relieved by applying cool compresses. The most frequent complication of any rash is a secondary bacterial infection, most often caused by excessive scratching. Call your doctor if any of the following symptoms are present:

- Temperature above 101 degrees
- Rash covering most of the body
- Rash getting worse instead of better
- Joint or muscle pain
- Blisters
- Pus or redness around the rash
- Red streaks on any limbs

Sore Throat

The majority of sore throats are caused by viruses, which cannot be helped by antibiotic treatment. (See Chapters 10 and 30.) However, all sore throats seen by a doctor need to be cultured for streptococcus (strep throat), which *does* warrant antibiotic treatment. Call your doctor if any of the following symptoms are present:

- Temperature above 101 degrees
- Pulse above 100 beats per minute
- Difficulty breathing
- Difficulty swallowing
- Skin rash
- Swollen glands under the jaw
- Earache or headache

Urinary Pain, Frequency or Blood

With any urinary complaints, the urine itself needs to be examined at the laboratory. Urinary issues tend to be more serious in men and children than in adult women. In females, they may be attributed to a treatable infection at least 50% of the time. For all urinary complaints, large fluid intake is advised (plain water is best). Call your doctor if any of the following symptoms are present:

- Fever (one degree elevation or higher)
- Severe pain
- Blood or pus in the urine
- Abdominal pain
- Itching

Vaginal Discharge or Irritation

Since there are a variety of causes for this type of irritation, this complaint needs to be seen in the doctor's office where a diagnosis can be made after microscopic evaluation. Do not douche for at least twenty-four hours before your examination.

Always Seek Medical Care *If*...

In addition to the alphabetical list already presented, be sure to seek medical advice if you have *any* of the following:

- Fever, *with no other symptoms*, that lasts more than one day
- Any recurrent symptoms you cannot tie to a specific cause
- Urinary symptoms of any kind in men or children
- Swelling anywhere, unless you are certain of its cause
- Any unexplained alteration of the function(s) of any part of the body
- Exposure to poisons
- A foreign body, anywhere
- Any injury that remains painful for more than seven days
- Chest pain associated with exercise
- Any of the known danger signs of cancer (change in bowel movements, sore that doesn't heal, unusual discharge or bleeding, thicknesses or lumps under the skin, indigestion or difficulty swallowing, changes in moles or warts, persistent cough or hoarseness)
- Any symptom that begins to affect your ability to concentrate, sleep or enjoy life

APPENDIX C

Your Medical Records

Important Health History

Your medical records are important! In fact, your medical records are the most powerful and effective instrument you have when it comes to managing and evaluating your own health care. They contain the history of your office visits, examinations, lab results, procedures and diagnoses from birth to death, having been added to and refined along the way. These records exist not only for the use and benefit of the physicians who examine you, but also for your own.

It's very important for patients to help build and polish their own medical records. Anything written in the record should be true, complete and acceptable to you. Nothing is gained by doctors writing something in your chart that they don't want you to see or know about. You also have the right to dispute what has been written. If you disagree with your doctor on some matter, request that he or she add a note in the record regarding the specifics of the disagreement. This would at least clarify the dispute for the next doctor.

You have the right to access and use your records in whatever way you choose. While it is highly appropriate to store them in the doctor's office, it is also wise to keep a continuously updated copy in your home for immediate reference. In fact, I do this with my own records and those of my family. With the possible exception of a psychiatrist, doctors have no right to withhold records from patients or their chosen next physicians for any reason. In fact, if any doctor attempts to do so, you have recourse via your local medical society to force release.

Abbreviations and Codes

In order to assist you in understanding what has been written in your records, what follows is a basic description of the abbreviations and codes most often used by physicians. This knowledge is also helpful when you have a written prescription to take to a pharmacy, so you can protect yourself from potentially dangerous human errors. Keep in mind that some medical codes change over time and eventually may no longer be applicable. Most libraries also have patient-friendly books on this topic.

Standard "SOAP" Notes

S = Subjective (what you tell the doctor)
O = Objective (findings of the physical examination)
A = Assessment (diagnosis)
P = Plan (course of action)

General

pt = patient
c/o = complains of
s/s = signs and symptoms
dx = diagnosis
FH = family history
OH = occupational history
hx = history of
abx = antibiotics
f/u = follow-up
c = with
s = without
hyper = high
hypo = low
L = left

R = right

B = bilateral

ROM = range of motion

Timing

a = before

p = after

q = every

BID = twice a day

TID = three times a day

QID = four times a day

QD = every day

QOD = every other day

PRN = as needed

QNS = enough to do the job

DC = discontinue

STAT = immediately

Other

CNS = central nervous system

TM = ear drum

N/V/D = nausea/vomiting/diarrhea

CBC = complete blood count

FUO = fever of unknown origin

FX = fracture

SOB = shortness of breath

Acknowledgments

for Walt Stoll, MD

William Harvey, Louis Pasteur, Joseph Lister, John Morgan, Ignaz Semmelweis, Horace Wells, Sir William Jenner and Sir Alexander Fleming are just a few of the many giants upon which the most valuable aspects of twentieth century conventional medicine have been based. Given that their views and discoveries were considered radical for their time, most of them were demonized and attacked unmercifully by their contemporaries.

Giants like Linus Pauling, PhD, Richard Passwater, PhD, Hans Selye, MD, Abram Hoffer, MD, PhD, Carlton Fredericks, PhD, Roger Williams, PhD, Samuel Hahnemann, MD, Andrew Still, MD, DO, Jeffrey Bland, PhD, Brugh Joy, MD, John Myers, MD, Ida Rolf, PhD, Harris Coulter, PhD, Paavo Airola, ND, Bernard Jensen, ND, Orion Truss, MD, Christopher Hills, PhD, Kenneth Pelletier, PhD, Robert Anderson, MD, Nathan Pritikin, Robert Becker, MD, Richard Gerber, MD and other forward-thinking individuals too numerous to mention have bravely opened the doors to a truly holistic vision of health care for the twenty-first century. Most of these medical visionaries and their followers have also been, and continue to be, just as viciously attacked by their contemporaries.[1] We owe them a debt of gratitude that can never be fully paid.

On a more personal note, I would like to thank my co-authoring partner, writer and editor, Kathleen M. Diehl. She possesses a real gift for writing and a true talent for putting complicated information into an easily understood form. Were it not for her professionalism and her years of research, dedication and diligence, this book would never have materialized. I would also like to thank publisher Jan DeCourtney for managing the publication, marketing and distribution aspects. Due to her tireless efforts, this book will be made available to the widest possible number of readers. Finally, I would like to thank my son, Bill Stoll, for his unwavering support as webmaster for "Ask Dr. Stoll" from its inception, without which none of my online endeavors would have been successful.[2]

Acknowledgments

for Kathleen M. Diehl

Being the unbelievably blessed mom that I am, I would like to begin by thanking my two wonderful sons, Shane and Eric, both of whom have shown incredible patience and tolerance with my incessant commands of "Shhh! Turn it down, I'm trying to write!" I am in awe of all the sacrifices they willingly made over the years in order to allow their noise-sensitive mother her quiet time for the research and writing of this book.

Many thanks also go to the various individuals who have taken the time to read chapters and offer their feedback and suggestions along the way, most notably publisher Jan DeCourtney, professional editor Barbara Munson and volunteer proofreaders Sheela Ayyagari, Angel R. Hayse, Bridget Hoy, William Mark, Kevin Diehl, Shane Diehl, John Marlow, Elane Marlow, Jarita Sadler and Anita Carnell Rowe. In addition, grateful acknowledgment is extended to our talented illustrator Debra M. Deutsch, page designer Marny K. Parkin, cover artist Tamara Dever and frontspiece consultants Diana Orr and Brenda Orr.

Last but not least, I would like to thank my co-author Walt Stoll, MD, both for opening up a whole new world in my understanding of health and dis-ease, and for entrusting me with the job of writing about his journey, his insights and his truths. Through the process of working closely with him on this book over the years, I have practically earned my own MD. His dedication to getting this valuable information out to as many people as possible is truly inspiring.

Notes

Foreword by Robert Anderson, MD

1. J. Lazarou, et al. "Incidence of Adverse Drug Reactions in Hospitalized Patients." *JAMA.* 279:1200–05, 1998. Article available online at: http://jama.ama-assn.org/cgi/content/full/279/15/1200?ijkey=F8guE.zA8WYTs/.

Sarah Loughran. "In Hospital Deaths from Medical Errors at 195,000 per Year USA" *Healthgrades.* August 9, 2004. Article available online at: http://www.medicalnewstoday.com/articles/11856.php.

2. S. Harvey Sklar, et al. "Herpes Zoster: The Treatment and Prevention of Neuralgia with Adenosine Monophosphate." *JAMA.* 253:1427–30, 1985. Article available online at: http://jama.ama-assn.org/cgi/content/abstract/253/10/1427/.

3. H.L. Bennett, PhD, et al. "Preoperative Instructions for Decreasing Bleeding During Spine Surgery." *Anesthesiology.* 65:A-245, 1986. Article available online at: http://journals.lww.com/anesthesiology/Citation/1986/09001/Preoperative_Instructions_for_Decreased_Bleeding.244.aspx.

See also: "Want Better Health? Use Your Head." *American Psychological Association.* December 15, 2003. Article available online at: http://www.apa.org/research/action/head.aspx.

Preface by Walt Stoll, MD

1. For the latest in DNA research, please visit the National Human Genome Research Institute at: http://www.genome.gov.

Introduction by Kathleen M. Diehl

1. Ask Dr. Stoll: Information About Combining Conventional & Alternative Medicine. http://www.askwaltstollmd.com.

Ask Dr. Stoll Bulletin Board. http://www.askwaltstollmd.com/wwwboard/wwwboard.html.

2. Walt Stoll, MD. *Saving Yourself From the Disease-Care Crisis.* Sunrise Health Coach, 1996.

Chapter 1. Health Care or *Disease* Care?

1. *See Chapter 1, Note 12 plus:*

Charles B. Inlander. *Medicine on Trial: The Appalling Story of Medical Ineptitude and the Arrogance That Overlooks It.* (Book of the Year: American Journal of Nursing 1989). Pantheon, 1989.

"Chronic Diseases and Health Promotion." *Centers for Disease Control and Prevention.* Article with 15 references available online at: http://www.cdc.gov/chronicdisease/overview/index.htm.

2. "The Pharmaceutical Fraud." *Dr. Rath Health Foundation.* Article available online at: http://www.nuremberg-tribunal.org/fraud/index.html.

3. The famous phrase "First, do no harm" likely came around 400 BC from *Of the Epidemics,* one of at least sixteen other important medical teachings authored by the ancient Greek physician, Hippocrates. In *Of the Epidemics,* Hippocrates states: "The physician must be able to tell the antecedents, know the present and foretell the future—must mediate these things, and have two special objects in view with regard to disease, namely, to do good or to *do no harm.*"

See also: G.E.R. Lloyd, editor. Translated by Chadwick and Mann. *Hippocratic Writings.* Penguin Classics, 1984.

N.S. Gill. "Is 'First Do No Harm' from the Hippocratic Oath? Myth Versus Fact." Article available online at: http://ancienthistory.about.com/od/greekmedicine/f/HippocraticOath.htm.

4. Francis Adams, translator. "Works" by Hippocrates. New York; Loeb. Volume I, 299–301.

5. A modern version of the Hippocratic Oath is available online at: http://primehcp.com/hippocrates.html.

6. The ancient Greek philosopher Democritus was the first well-known proponent of the atomistic way of thinking, later bolstered by Descartes, the "Father of Modern Philosophy."

See also: Martin J. Walker. *Dirty Medicine: Science, Big Business, and the Assault on Natural Health Care.* Slingshot Publications, 1993.

7. Alyn Brodsky. *Benjamin Rush: Patriot and Physician.* Truman Talley Books, 2004.

8. Mark Silverman, et al., editors. *The Quotable Osler.* Revised paperback edition. American College of Physicians, 2007.

9. Richard Grossinger. *Planet Medicine: Origins* and *Planet Medicine: Modalities.* North Atlantic Books, revised ed., 2001–2003.

Harris L. Coulter. *Divided Legacy Volumes I–IV.* Wehawken Book Co. and North Atlantic Books, 1975–1994.

10. Dean Black, PhD. *Pigs in the Dirt: How a Little Common Sense Can Help Resolve the HealthCare Mess.* Tapestry Press, 1993.

Dean Black, PhD. *Health at the Crossroads: Exploring the Conflict Between Natural Healing and Conventional Medicine.* Tapestry Press, 1988.

11. Andrew Zimmerman-Jones. "Wave-Particle Duality." Article available online at: http://physics.about.com/od/lightoptics/a/waveparticle.htm.

12. Walt's years of comprehensive holistic health knowledge was derived from his personal experiences as an MD as well as from the following core group of his favorite resources:

Robert Anderson, MD. *Dr. Robert Anderson's Comprehensive Guide to Wellness Medicine.* Keats Publishers, 1993. (2,141 references.)

Dean Black, PhD. *Health at the Crossroads: Exploring the Conflict Between Natural Healing and Conventional Medicine.* Tapestry Press, 1988.

Dean Black, PhD. *Pigs in the Dirt: How a Little Common Sense Can Help Resolve the Health Care Mess.* Tapestry Press, 1993.

James P. Carter. *Racketeering in Medicine: The Suppression of Alternatives.* Hampton Roads, 1992.

Harris L. Coulter. *Divided Legacy Volumes I–IV.* Wehawken Book Co. and North Atlantic Books, 1975–1994.

Richard Grossinger. *Planet Medicine: Origins,* and *Planet Medicine: Modalities.* North Atlantic Books, revised ed., 2001–2003.

Jane Heimlich. *What Your Doctor Won't Tell You: The Complete Guide to the Latest in Alternative Medicine.* Harper Paperbacks, 1990.

Joseph P. Lisa. *The Assault on Medical Freedom.* Hampton Roads, 1994.

Joseph P. Lisa. *The Great Medical Monopoly Wars.* International Institute of Natural Health Sciences, 1986.

Dr. Kenneth R. Pelletier. *Mind as Healer, Mind as Slayer.* Delta, 1978. An updated and revised edition is forthcoming.

Hugh Riordan, MD. *Medical Mavericks, Volumes I, II and III.* Biocommunications Press, 1988–90. To order call: 800-447-7276.

Hans Selye, MD. *The Stress of Life.* McGraw/Hill, 1956. Revised and reprinted in 1984.

Martin J. Walker. *Dirty Medicine: Science, Big Business, and the Assault on Natural Health Care.* Slingshot Publications, 1993.

Chapter 2. From Conventional to Holistic: How I Lost My License

1. For more information on Silva Mind Training, visit The Silva Method website: http://www.silvamethod.com. (800)545-6463.

2. Walt's "New Patient Handbook" was first published in 1976 with new editions 1977, 1978, 1979, 1980, 1981, 1984, 1986 and 1988.

3. Mary Chamberlain. "Pay the Doctor Only if He Keeps You Well." Article available online at: http://www.saratoga.com/healing-arts/2009/05/the-beauty-of-chinese-medicine.html.

4. Due to the AMA's longstanding pattern of harassment, the American Association for Health Freedom has written *A Practitioner's Guide to Protecting Your License*

and Your Practice from Medical Board and Other Government Action. Available to Alliance for Natural Health (ANH-USA) members on http://www.anh-usa.org/practitioner/.

Additional information at: http://thehealthfreedom.blogspot.com/2008/04/integrative-medicine-practitioners-are.html.

5. Alexis Black. "Unnecessary Surgery Exposed! Why 60% of All Surgeries Are Medically Unjustified and How Surgeons Exploit Patients to Generate Profits." *Natural News*. Article available online at: http://www.naturalnews.com/012291.html.

See also: Mark Hyman, MD and Mark Liponis. *Ultraprevention: The 6-Week Plan That Will Make You Healthy for Life*. Scribner, 2003.

Burton Goldberg. *Heart Disease, Stroke and High Blood Pressure: An Alternative Medicine Guide*. Alternativemedicine.com Books, 1998.

6. Ask Dr. Stoll: Information About Combining Conventional & Alternative Medicine. http://www.askwaltstollmd.com.

Ask Dr. Stoll Bulletin Board. http://www.askwaltstollmd.com/wwwboard/wwwboard.html.

Walt Stoll, MD. *Saving Yourself From the Disease-Care Crisis*. Sunrise Health Coach Publications, 1996.

Walt Stoll, MD and Jan DeCourtney, CMT. *Recapture Your Health: A Step-By-Step Program to Reverse Chronic Symptoms and Create Lasting Wellness*. Sunrise Health Coach Publications, 2006.

Chapter 3. The Conventional Medical Monopoly

1. *See Chapter 1, Note 12.*

2. A.R. Marth. "A History of the American Medical Association (AMA)." *Helium: Where Knowledge Rules*. Article available online at: http://www.helium.com/items/267216-a-history-of-the-american-medical-association-ama/.

Llewellyn H. Rockwell Jr. "The American Medical Association: A Sordid History." *Health E-Living News*. Article available online at: http://www.healthe-livingnews.com/articles/american_medical_association_sorbid_history.html.

For more information, read: Educate Yourself: Forbidden Cures at: http://www.educate-yourself.org.

3. Llewellyn H. Rockwell Jr. as cited in *Healing Beyond the Body: Medicine and the Infinite Reach of the Mind* by Larry Dossey, MD. Shambhala, 2001.

4. William James as cited in *Health Education: A Cognitive-Behavioral Approach* by Donald A. Read, PhD. Jones and Bartlett Publishers, 1996.

William James as cited in *Patient Power: Solving America's Health Care Crisis* by John C. Goodman and Gerald L. Musgrave. Cato Institute, 1992.

For more information about William James see: http://en.wikipedia.org/wiki/William_James/.

5. John C. Goodman, and Gerald L. Musgrave. *Patient Power: Solving America's Health Care Crisis.* Cato Institute, 1992.

6. *See Chapter 3, Note 2* plus:

Llewellyn H. Rockwell Jr. "Medical Control, Medical Corruption." *LewRockwell.com.* Article available online at: http://www.lewrockwell.com/rockwell/medical.html.

7. Ibid. *See also: Chapter 1, Note 12.*

8. Ken Adachi. "U.S. Judge Finds Medical Group Conspired Against Chiropractors." *The New York Times.* August 29, 1987. Article available online at: www.nytimes.com/1987/08/29/us/us-judge-finds-medical-group-conspired-against-chiropractors.html?pagewanted=1/.

9. Article originally published in *Alternative Medicine Digest,* Issue 11. April, 1996. Available through the Institute for Health Freedom. For more information, visit their website at: http://www.forhealthfreedom.org.

10. Gary Null, PhD, et al. *Death by Medicine,* 2003. Full report available online at: http://www.whale.to/a/null9.html.

11. David Pimentel. "Erosion and Malnutrition." *Science.* February 24, 1995.

12. E. Pennisi. "Biodiversity Helps Keep Ecosystems Healthy." *Science News.* February 5, 1994. Article available online at: http://findarticles.com/p/articles/mi_m1200/is_n6_v145/ai_14818126/.

Kathy A. Fackelman. "Reassessing Pesticides' Value." *Science News.* 144:5, page 79. January 29, 1994.

For more information on the dangers of environmental agents, contact:

1) The Chemical Injury Information Network (CIIN). http://ciin.org. (406)547-2255.

2) Human Ecology Action League (HEAL). http://www.healnatl.org. (770)389-4519.

13. Gary Null, PhD, et al. *Death by Medicine.* 2003. According to this report, "By 1995, drug companies had tripled the amount of money allotted to direct advertising of prescription drugs to consumers. The majority of the money is spent on seductive television ads. From 1996 to 2000, spending rose from $791 million to nearly $2.5 billion. [This] only represents 15% of the total pharmaceutical advertising budget." Full report available online at: http://www.whale.to/a/null9.html.

See also: DOC News. Volume 3, Number 2, p. 13. February 1, 2006.

Melody Petersen. *Our Daily Meds: How the Pharmaceutical Companies Transformed Themselves into Slick Marketing Machines and Hooked the Nation on Prescription Drugs.* Reprinted by Picador, 2009.

M.B. Rosenthal, et al. "Promotion of Prescription Drugs to Consumers." *New England Journal of Medicine.* 346(7):498–505, 2/14/02.

C.B. Sufrin and J.S. Ross. "Pharmaceutical Industry Marketing: Understanding Its Impact on Women's Health." *Obstetrical & Gynecological Survey.* 63 (9):585–96. September, 2008.

14. Stanley Wohl, MD. *The Medical Industrial Complex.* Harmony Books, 1984.

John Abramson, MD. *Overdosed America: The Broken Promise of American Medicine.* 3rd edition. Harper Perennial, 2008.

Marcia Angell, MD. *The Truth About the Drug Companies: How They Deceive Us and What to Do About It.* Random House Trade Paperbacks, 2005.

Jacky Law. *Big Pharma: Exposing the Global Healthcare Agenda.* Basic Books, 2006.

Ray Moynihan and Alan Cassels. *Selling Sickness: How the World's Biggest Pharmaceutical Companies Are Turning Us All into Patients.* Nation Books, 2006.

15. *See Chapter 1, Note 12 plus:*

M. Winnick. "Nutritional Education in Medical Schools." *American Journal of Clinical Nutrition.* 58: 825–27. 1993.

M. Zimmerman and N. Kretchmer. "Isn't It Time to Teach Nutrition to Medical Students?" *American Journal of Clinical Nutrition.* 58: 828–29. 1993.

16. Robert Mendelsohn, MD. *Confessions of a Medical Heretic.* Warner Books, 1987.

17. "The Use of Complementary and Alternative Medicine in the United States." National Center for Complementary and Alternative Medicine (NCCAM). Article available online at: http://nccam.nih.gov/news/camstats/2007/camsurvey_fs1.htm.

See also: "Alternative Medicine (a Three-Part Series)." *Consumer Reports.* January, March, June 1994.

18. Alan Bensoussan and George Lewith. "Complementary Medicine Research in Australia: a Strategy for the Future." *Medical Journal of Australia (MJA).* 181(6):331–33, 2004.

Chapter 4. Beyond Disease Care

1. For more information on the Human Genome Project, please visit the National Human Genome Research Institute at: http://www.genome.gov.

2. Roger J. Williams, PhD. *Biochemical Individuality: The Key to Understanding What Shapes Your Health.* Keats Publishing, 1998.

Roger J. Williams, PhD. *The Wonderful World Within You.* Bio-Communications Press, 1998.

For a bio of Roger Williams, please see: http://bioinst.cm.utexas.edu/williams/.

3. *Functional Medicine Update* (FMU). 1981–Present.

4. E. Arias, et al. "Deaths: Preliminary Data for 2001." *CDC National Vital Statistics Reports.* 51:5, March 14, 2003. Article available online at: http://www.cdc.gov/nchs/data/nvsr/nvsr51/nvsr51_05.pdf/.

Gary Null, PhD. et al. *Death by Medicine.* 2003. Full report available online at: http://www.whale.to/a/null9.html.

According to Nancy Dubler in *Ethics on Call: How to Take Charge of Life-and-Death Choices in Today's Health Care System.* Vintage, 1993, "In 1990, we spent $666 million on health care—$2,664 for every man, woman and child. Yet for those billions of dollars, we rank 16th in life expectancy, 23rd in infant mortality and 24th in the percentage of normal birth-weight babies—behind Bulgaria, the Soviet Union and Hong Kong."

According to "Why Not the Best? Results from the National Scorecard on U.S. Health System Performance." The Commonwealth Fund Commission on a High Performance Health System, 2008, "the U.S. now ranks last out of 19 countries on a measure of mortality amenable to medical care, falling from 15th as other countries raised the bar ... Performance of measures of health system efficiency remains especially low, with the U.S. scoring 53 out of 100 on measures gauging inappropriate, wasteful or fragmented care, avoiding hospitalizations, variation in quality and costs, administrative costs and use of information technology." Article available online at: http://www.commonwealthfund.org/publications/publications_show.htm?doc_id=692682/.

See also: Sepp Hasslberger. "Medical System Is Leading Cause of Death and Injury in U.S." Article available online at: http://www.newmediaexplorer.org/sepp/2003/10/29/medical_system_is_leading_cause_of_death_and_injury_in_us.htm.

5. "Is Your Doctor Board Certified? Does It Matter?" *Consumer's Checkbook*. Article available online at: http://www.checkbook.org/boardcert/.

6. The Serenity Prayer was written by theologian Reinhold Niebuhr and is frequently recited in 12-Step programs such as Alcoholics Anonymous.

Chapter 5. Modern Medical Interpretation of Stress

1. Global 2000 U.S. Study. *The Global 2000 Report to the President: Entering the 21st Century*. University of Michigan Library, 1980.

2. William Arntz, et al. *What the Bleep Do We Know!? Discovering the Endless Possibilities for Altering Your Everyday Reality*. HCI/MTI edition, 2007. *See also: What the Bleep Do We Know!?* movie.

Rhonda Byrne. *The Secret*. Atria Books/Beyond Words, 2006. *See also: The Secret* movie.

Deepak Chopra, MD. *Quantum Healing: Exploring the Frontiers of Mind-Body Medicine*. Bantam, 1990.

Dr. Wayne Dyer. *Manifest Your Destiny: Nine Principles for Getting Everything You Want*. Harper Collins, 1997.

Esther and Jerry Hicks. *The Law of Attraction: The Basics of the Teachings of Abraham*. Hay House, 2006.

For assistance with the challenges that may arise during the spiritual awakening process, contact:

1) Spiritual Emergence Network (SEN). http://www.spiritualemeergence.info/. (415)453-1106.

2) Edgar Cayce's A.R.E. Association for Research and Enlightenment. http://www.edgarcayce.org/. (800)333-4499.

3) Kathleen M. Diehl's spiritual coaching service. http://kathleendiehl.com/askme.htm.

3. Dr. Kenneth R. Pelletier. *Mind as Healer, Mind as Slayer*. Delta, 1978. Updated and revised edition is forthcoming.

4. Hans Selye, MD. *The Stress of Life*. McGraw/Hill, 1956. Revised and reprinted in 1984.

Herbert Benson, MD. *The Relaxation Response*. G.K. Hall, 1976. This #1 best-seller was updated, expanded, reprinted edition with co-author Miriam Z. Klipper in 2000 by Harper Paperbacks.

Dr. Kenneth R. Pelletier. *Mind as Healer, Mind as Slayer*. Delta, 1978. Updated and revised edition is forthcoming.

5. Serdar Z. Elgun (preparer). "Introduction to Industrial Hygiene." Article available online at: http://info.lu.farmingdale.edu/depts/met/ind310/indhygintro.html.

6. "Trade Secrets: A Moyers Report." In this 90-minute special presented on PBS television, Bill Moyers explained the hidden dangers of the chemical industry and exposing the political games being played with our lives. He describes a "campaign to limit the regulation of toxic chemicals and any liability for their effects, at the same time that the companies work to withhold vital information about the risks from workers, the government and the public." For more information see: http://www.pbs.org/tradesecrets/program/overview.html.

7. *See Chapter 1, Note 12*. Although the exact reference for this particular study has been lost, Dr. Stoll has been quoting these figures for several years based on his ongoing study and best recollection.

8. Visit ACE: The Alliance for a Clean Environment at: http://www.acereport.org/children2.html.

9. A-P Wire Service, 2001.

10. "Are Genetically Modified Foods Behind the Increase in Food Allergies?" *The Nontoxic Times Newsletter*. Article available online at: https://www.achooallergy.com/blog/genetically-modified-foods/Default.asp.

11. Dr. George Carlo and Martin Schram. *Cell Phones: Invisible Hazards in the Wireless Age*. Carroll & Graf, 2002.

For additional information, please visit the following URLs:

1) http://www.foxnews.com/story/0,2933,569465,00.html.

2) http://www.medicalnewstoday.com/articles/161960.php.

3) http://environment.about.com/b/2009/03/17/study-finds-cell-phones-increase-brain-cancer-risks-in-children.htm.

12. Samuel Maguire-Boyle and Andrew R. Barron. "Connections: Theory of a Superconducting Quantum Interfering Device (SQUID)." *Connections*. Article available online at: http://cnx.org/content/m22750/1.3/.

Stephanie Relfe. "Stress from Electromagnetic and Ionizing Radiation: A Major Cause of Health Problems and Emotional Stress." *Health, Wealth & Happiness*. Chart available online at: www.relfe.com/electromagnetic.html.

"Electromagnetic Stress. *The Healthy House, Ltd*. Article available online at: http://www.healthy-house.co.uk/allergy/electromagnetic_stress.php.

13. Andrew Weil, MD. *8 Weeks to Optimum Health: A Proven Program for Taking Full Advantage of Your Body's Natural Healing Power.* Ballantine Books, 2007.

Andrew Weil, MD *Spontaneous Healing: How to Discover and Embrace Your Body's Natural Ability to Maintain and Heal Itself.* Ballantine Books, 2000.

14. Paul Brodeur. *Currents of Death: The Attempt to Cover Up the Threat to Your Health.* Simon and Schuster, 1989.

Cyril W. Smith and Simon Best. *Electromagnetic Man: Health & Hazard in the Electrical Environment.* Martin's Press, Inc., 1989.

F. Hollwich. *The Influence of Ocular Light Perception on Metabolism in Man and Animal.* Translated by Hunter and Hildegarde Hannum. Springer-Verlag, 1979.

"Another Way EMFs Might Harm Tissues." *Science News.* 145:8, p. 127. February 19, 1994.

William Hendee, MD and John C. Boteler, PhD. "The Question of Health Effects From Exposure to Electromagnetic Fields." *Health Physics.* 66:127–136, 1994.

B. Hileman. "Health Effects of Electromagnetic Fields Remain Unresolved." *Chemical and Engineering News.* pp. 15–29. November, 1993.

15. Martin L. Pall, PhD. *Explaining Unexplained Illnesses: Disease Paradigm for Chronic Fatigue Syndrome, Multiple Chemical Sensitivity, Fibromyalgia, Post-Traumatic Stress Disorder and Gulf War Syndrome.* Informa Health Care, 2007.

John Travis, MD, MPH and Regina Ryan. *Wellness, Small Changes.* 10 Speed Press, 1991.

John Travis, MD. *Wellness Workbook.* 10 Speed Press, 1988.

Martin J. Walker. *Dirty Medicine: Science, Big Business, and the Assault on Natural Health Care.* Slingshot Publications, 1993.

16. Dr. Kenneth R. Pelletier. *Mind as Healer, Mind as Slayer.* Delta, 1978. Updated and revised edition is forthcoming.

Hans Selye, MD. *The Stress of Life.* McGraw/Hill, 1956. Revised and reprinted in 1984.

17. Dr. Stoll viewed this on CNN, February 1995.

18. Jason Serinus, editor. *Psychoimmunity and the Healing Process.* Celestial Arts, 1986.

E. Pennisi and K.A. Fackelmann. "HIV Toll: Over a Billion White Cells a Day." *Science News.* p 21, January 14, 1995.

M.S. Kapemba, et al. "Altered Cell Intestinal Permeability Associated with Diarrhea in HIV-Positive Individuals." *Clinical Science.* 81:327, 1992.

Robin Marantz Henig. *A Dancing Matrix: Voyages Along a Viral Frontier.* Knopf. 1993.

19. As reported at the annual international meeting of clinical ecologists in Dallas in May 1985.

Chapter 6. Stored Stress-Effect and the Hypothalamus

1. Vic Braden. *Vic Braden's Mental Tennis: How to Psyche Yourself to a Winning Game.* Little, Brown & Co. 1994.

2. Dr. Kenneth R. Pelletier. *Mind as Healer, Mind as Slayer*. Delta, 1978. Updated and revised edition is forthcoming.

3. Adapted from R.M. Yerkes, J.D. Dodson. "The Relation of Strength of Stimulus to Rapidity of Habit Formation." *Journal of Comparative Neurology and Psychology*. 18(5) 459–82. Reprinted with permission of Robert Anderson, MD A Dictionary of Psychology. Oxford University Press, 2001.

"Yerkes-Dodson Law." ChangingMinds.org. Article available online at: http://changingminds.org/explanations/motivation/yerkes-dodson.htm.

4. Hans Selye, MD. *The Stress of Life*. McGraw/Hill, 1956. Revised and reprinted in 1984.

5. Davis, et al. *The Relaxation & Stress Reduction Workbook*. 6th edition. New Harbinger Publications, 2008.

Rosie Speigel. *Bodies, Health and Consciousness: A Guide to Living Successfully in Your Body Through Rolfing and Yoga*. S R G Publishing, 1994.

Don Johnson. *The Protean Body: A Rolfer's View of Human Flexibility*. Harper Collins, 1977.

The Rolf Institute of Structural Integration. http://www.rolf.org. (303)449-5903.

See also: Davis, et al. *The Relaxation & Stress Reduction Workbook*. 6th edition. New Harbinger Publications, 2008.

Roger Golton. *The Owner's Guide to the Body: How to Have a Perfectly Tuned Body and Mind*. Thorsons, 1999.

Chapter 7. Leaky Gut Syndrome

1. Genova Diagnostics, Intestinal Permeability Assessment. For more information or to order this test, please visit: http://www.genovadiagnostics.com/index.php?option=com_gpanel&Itemid=2&task=view&nav=test&id=18/.

2. Elizabeth Lipski. *Leaky Gut Syndrome: What to Do About a Health Threat that Can Cause Arthritis, Allergies, and a Host of Other Illnesses*. McGraw-Hill, 1998.

See also: R. Troncone, et al. "Increased Intestinal Sugar Permeability After Challenge in Children with Cow's Milk Allergy or Intolerance." *Allergy*. 49:142–6, 1994.

R.E. Tepper, et al. "Intestinal Permeability in Patients Infected with Human Immunodeficiency Virus." *American Journal of Gastroenterology*. 89:878, 1994.

R. Paganelli, et al. "Intestinal Permeability in Patients with Chronic Urticaria-angioedema with and without Arthralgia." *Annals of Allergy*. 66:181–4, 1991.

O. Martinez-Gonzalez, et al. "Intestinal Permeability in Patients Infected with Ankylosing Spondylitis and Their Healthy Relatives." *British Journal of Rheumatology*. 333:644–7, 1994.

3. Ibid. *See also*: A. Vojdani, et al. "Immune Response to Dietary Proteins, Gliadin and Cerebellar Peptides in Children with Autism." *Nutritional Neuroscience*. 7:3, 151–161. June, 2004.

4. "Conversion of Food-Borne Heterocyclic Amine Carcinogens." *National Cancer Institute*. 6:5, 1994.

5. Ibid. *See also:* D.R. Dantzkler. "The Gastrointestinal Tract: The Canary of the Body?" *Journal of the American Medical Association*. 270:1247–8, 1993.

For information on mercury toxicity from dental amalgams, contact Huggins Applied Healing at: http://www.hugginsappliedhealing.com/. (866)948-4638.

6. Michael Gershon, MD. *The Second Brain: A Groundbreaking New Understanding of Nervous Disorders of the Stomach and Intestine*. HarperCollins, 1999.

Elizabeth Lipski. *Leaky Gut Syndrome: What to Do About a Health Threat That Can Cause Arthritis, Allergies, and a Host of Other Illnesses*. McGraw-Hill, 1998.

7. For more information, visit the American Dysautonomia Institute at: http://www.adiwebsite.org/index2.html.

8. Dr. Kenneth R. Pelletier. *Mind as Healer, Mind as Slayer*. Delta, 1978. Updated and revised edition is forthcoming.

See also: Jim Robbins. *A Symphony in the Brain: The Evolution of the New Brain Wave Biofeedback*. Revised edition. Grove Press, 2008.

Chapter 8: Candida-Related Syndrome

1. *For more information on Candida-Related Syndrome, consult the following resources:*

William G. Crook, MD. *The Yeast Connection: A Medical Breakthrough*. Updated and revised. Vintage Books, 1986.

William G. Crook, MD. *The Yeast Connection Handbook*. Square One Publishers, 1999.

Jeanne M. Martin and Rona P. Zoltan, MD. *Complete Candida Yeast Guidebook: Everything You Need to Know About Prevention, Treatment and Diet*. Revised 2nd edition. Three Rivers Press, 2000.

John P. Trowbridge, MD and Morton Walker. *The Yeast Syndrome: How to Help Your Doctor Identify & Treat the Real Cause of Your Yeast-Related Illness*. Bantam Books. 1986.

Orian C. Truss, MD. *The Missing Diagnosis: Chronic Candidiasis*. Missing Diagnosis, 1985.

Orian C. Truss, MD. *The Missing Diagnosis II*. Published by the author, 2009.

2. Ibid.

3. Genova Diagnostics (formerly Great Smokies Diagnostic Labs GDSL). 63 Zillicoa Street, Asheville, NC 28801. (800)522-4762. http://www.gdx.net.

Meridian Valley Lab. 801 SW 16th Street #126, Renton, WA 98055. (425)271-8689. http://www.meridianvalleylab.com.

Chapter 9: Allergy and Hypersensitivity

1. NBC News, January 1995.

See also: "CDC Fast Facts A–Z," Vital Health Statistics, 2003 (1 in 5).

Rachel Rettner. "Americans Sneeze More As Allergies Mysteriously Increase." *LiveScience*, March 2010. Article available online at: http://www.livescience.com/health/allergy-increase-100326.html.

2. Theron Randolph, MD and Ralph W. Moss, PhD. *An Alternative Approach to Allergies: The New Field of Clinical Ecology Unravels the Environmental Causes of Mental and Physical Ills.* Harper Perennial, 1990.

Theron Randolph, MD. *Environmental Medicine: Beginnings & Bibliographies of Clinical Ecology.* Clinical Ecology Publications. 1987.

Information on clinical ecology and Theron Randolph, MD can be found online at: http://www.methodsofhealing.com/Types_of_Healing/clinical-ecology/.

To find the nearest clinical ecologist, contact The American Academy of Environmental Medicine in Wichita, KS. http://www.aaemonline.org/. (316)684-5500.

3. Gary Null, PhD. *Nutrition and the Mind.* Seven Stories Press, 2003.

William Philpott, MD. *Brain Allergies: The Psychonutrient and Magnetic Connections.* Keats, 1980. Revised and reprinted 2nd edition by McGraw-Hill, 2000.

Alexander Schauss, PhD. *Diet, Crime and Delinquency: A New Breakthrough to Crime Control.* Parker House Enterprises, 1981.

David Sheinkin, MD and Michael Schachter, MD. *Food, Mind and Mood.* (formerly titled, *The Food Connection.*) Warner Books, 1987.

4. Theron Randolph, MD and Ralph W. Moss, PhD. *An Alternative Approach to Allergies: The New Field of Clinical Ecology Unravels the Environmental Causes of Mental and Physical Ills.* Harper Perennial, 1990.

Theron Randolph, MD. *Environmental Medicine: Beginnings & Bibliographies of Clinical Ecology.* Clinical Ecology Publications. 1987.

See also: Michael Gershon, MD. *The Second Brain: A Groundbreaking New Understanding of Nervous Disorders of the Stomach and Intestine.* HarperCollins, 1999.

5. Ibid.

6. Lisa Lewis, PhD. *Special Diets for Special Kids.* Future Horizons. 1998.

Lisa Lewis, PhD. *Special Diets for Special Kids, Two.* Future Horizons, 2001.

See also: Applied Kinesiology for Food Allergies: http://www.altmd.com/Articles/Applied-Kinesiology-for-Food-Allergies/.

Opioid Effect of Gluten & Casein: http://www.greatplainslaboratory.com/home/eng/peptide.asp.

Autism and Leaky Gut Syndrome: http://www.autism.com/families/diet/leakygut.htm.

Chapter 10: Recurrent Colds and Flu

1. Arthur C. Guyton, MD and John E. Hall, PhD. *Human Physiology and Mechanisms of Disease.* Saunders, 1996.

2. *Clinical Pediatrics.* 2:3, 119–121, 1963. DOI: 10.1177/000992286300200304.

3. Donald W. Miller Jr., MD. "Avoid Flu Shots, Take Vitamin D Instead." *American Journal of Clinical Nutrition*. 84:694–97, 2006.

Adit A. Ginde, et al. "Association Between Serum 25-Hydroxyvitamin D Level and Upper Respiratory Tract Infection in the Third National Health and Nutrition Examination Survey." *Archives of Internal Medicine*. 169(4):384. DOI: 10.1001/archinternmed.2008.560.

"Vitamin D Deficiency May Increase Risk of Colds, Flu." *Science Daily*. February 4, 2009.

4. Mike Adams, editor. "Sunscreen Use Actually Causes Cancer, It Doesn't Prevent It, Says Exhaustive Scientific Research." *Natural News*. July 5, 2004. Article available online at: http://www.naturalnews.com/001264.html.

"Sunscreen Causes Cancer!" *HolisticAnswers.com*. May 30, 2008. Article available online at: http://www.holisticanswers.org/?p=303/.

5. *See Chapter 10, Note 3.*

6. Stephen Langer. "When It Comes to Vitamins, 'Cs' Make the Grade." *Better Nutrition*. December, 1996.

Frank Murray. "Vitamin C Gets Even Better." Better Nutrition, 1990. Article available online at: http://findarticles.com/p/articles/mi_m0860/is_n3_v51/ai_7051810/.

Phyllis A. Balch, CNC. *Prescription for Nutritional Healing, 4th edition: A Practical A-to-Z Reference to Drug-Free Remedies Using Vitamins, Minerals, Herbs & Food Supplements*. Avery Trade, 2006.

7. "Cold-Eeze." The Quigley Corporation. Doylestown, PA. http://www.coldeeze.com/.

See also: Zicam Product Research. http://www.zicam.com/products/research/.

Godfrey et al. *Journal of International Medical Research*. 20:3. June, 1992.

Mossad et al. *Annals of Internal Medicine*. 125:2. July 15, 1996.

8. For information on nasal saline irrigation and Neti pots, visit: http://www.webmd.com/allergies/sinus-pain-pressure-9/neti-pots/.

9. Greg Ciola. "Flu Shot Dangers Far Outweigh Benefits." December 16, 2006. Article available online at: http://www.newswithviews.com/Ciola/greg.htm.

10. For information about the potential side-effects and dangers of the new Gardasil vaccine, including documented deaths and injuries, see the following websites:
1) http://naturalhealthnews.blogspot.com/2009/03/gardasil-death-and-danger-update.html.
2) http://homeopathyforwomen.org/gardasil_vaccine.htm.
3) http://truthaboutgardasil.org.
4) http://kdka.com/health/gardasil.danger.paralysis.2.765507.html.

11. To the best of Dr. Stoll's recollection, these facts are derived from what is known as the *Materia Medica*, denoting the collected body of medical knowledge over time.

12. Blair Justice, PhD. *Who Gets Sick (Thinking and Health)*. Peak Press, 1987.

Chapter 11: Recurrent Ear Infections

1. Erdem I. Cantekin, PhD, et al. "Antimicrobial Therapy for Otitis Media with Effusion." *JAMA*. 266(23):3309–17, 1991.

See also: "Ear Infections, Over-Treated?" February 15, 2008. Article available online at: http://www.diseaseproof.com/archives/ear-infections-ear-infections-overtreated.html.

Lists of published articles about antibiotics and ear infections can be found on this website: http://www.eardoc.info/news/antibiotics-are-really-bad-solution-for-ear-infections/.

2. *See Chapter 9, Note 6.*

3. Ian D. Coulter, PhD. "Efficacy and Risks of Chiropractic Manipulation: What Does the Evidence Suggest?" *Integrative Medicine*. 1:61–66, 1998.

Joan M. Fallon, DC. "The Role of the Chiropractic Adjustment in the Care and Treatment of 332 Children with Otitis Media." *Journal of Clinical Chiropractic Pediatrics*. 2(2): 167–183, 1997.

R.M. Froehl. "Ear Infection: A Retrospective Study Examining Improvement from Chiropractic Care and Analyzing for Influencing Factors." *Journal of Manipulative and Physiological Therapeutics*. 19(3):169–77. March–April, 1996.

Jane Sheppard. "Chiropractic for Chronic Ear Infections." *Healthy Child*. Article available online at: http://www.healthychild.com/chiropractic/chiropractic-for-chronic-ear-infections/.

"Chiropractic Approach to Ear Infections." *American Chiropractic Association*. Article available online at: http://www.acatoday.org/content_css.cfm?CID=69/.

Chapter 12: Recurrent Headaches

1. Meyer B. Marks, MD. "Physical Signs of Allergy of the Respiratory Tract in Children." *Annals of Allergy*. 25:310. June, 1967.

2. Andrew P. Jones, MD. "The Migraine Aura—Tricks from the Brain." January, 2010. Article available online at: http://www.articlesbase.com/diseases-and-conditions-articles/the-migraine-aura-tricks-from-the-brain-62657.html.

3. "Caffeine and Headache." National Headache Foundation. Article available online at: http://www.headaches.org/educational_modules/caffeine/fast.html.

Melissa C. Stoppler, MD. "Migraine Headache." Medicinenet. Article available online at: http://www.medicinenet.com/migraine_headache/page3.htm.

4. *See Chapter 6, Note 5 plus:*

For information on Hellerwork, visit Hellerwork Structural Integration at: http://hellerwork.com/.

Steven Shafarman. *Awareness Heals: The Feldenkrais Method for Dynamic Health*. Da Capo Press, 1997.

Michael J. Gelb. *Body Learning: An Introduction to the Alexander Technique*. Henry Holt & Co., 1981.

Chapter 13: Endocrine Disorders

1. Lawrence Foss. *The Second Medical Revolution: From Biomedicine to Infomedicine*. Shambhala, 1988.

`2. Dr. Kenneth R. Pelletier. *Mind as Healer, Mind as Slayer*. Delta, 1978. Updated and revised edition is forthcoming.

3. Information on Dr. Ghent's study on Lugol's can be obtained from Queen's University at Kingston, Ontario.

See also Chapter 13, Note 4 and: John A. Myers, MD and Karl H. Schutte, PhD. *Metabolic Aspects of Health: Nutritional Elements in Health and Disease*. Discovery Press, 1979.

4. David Brownstein, MD. *Iodine: Why You Need It, Why You Can't Live Without It*. 4th edition. Medical Alternative Press, 2009.

Also visit *The Iodine Group*. http://www.iodine4health.com/disease/disease.htm.

5. P.J. Rosch. "Stressful Life Events and Graves' Disease." *Lancet*. 342:566–7, 1993.

6. Ivan Illich. *Limits to Medicine: Medical Nemesis, the Expropriation of Health*. Marion Boyars Publishers, Ltd. 2000.

Chapter 14: Vascular Disorders

1. "What Are the AHA Blood Pressure Guidelines?" See: http://www.livestrong.com/article/104062-aha-blood-pressure-guidelines/.

"Your High Blood Pressure Questions Answered: Guidelines Lowered." See: http://www.americanheart.org/presenter.jhtml?identifier=3025147/.

A medical definition of hypertension can be found here: http://medical-dictionary.thefreedictionary.com/hypertension/.

2. Nathan Pritikin. *The Pritikin Program for Diet & Exercise*. Originally published by Grosset & Dunlap, 1979. Many reprintings since.

Visit the Pritikin Longevity Center at: http://www.pritikin.com/index.php?option=com_content&view=category&layout=blog&id=137&Itemid=123/.

3. Dean Ornish. *The Ornish Plan for Reversing Heart Disease*. HarperCollins, 1992. Reprinted as *Dr. Dean Ornish's Program for Reversing Heart Disease: The Only System Scientifically Proven to Reverse Heart Disease Without Drugs or Surgery*. Ballantine Books, 2008.

4. Elmer M. Cranton, MD. *A Textbook on EDTA Chelation Therapy*. 2nd Edition. Hampton Roads. 2001.

Elmer M. Cranton, MD. *Bypassing Bypass*. Medex Publishers, 1992. Reprinted as *Bypassing Bypass Surgery*. Hampton Roads, 2001.

Bruce W. Halstead, MD and Theodore C. Rozema. *The Scientific Basis of EDTA Chelation Therapy*. 2nd edition. TRC Publishing, 1997.

To find local chelating physicians, contact the American College for Advancement in Medicine (ACAM) at: www.acamnet.org. (800)532-3688.

5. Ibid.

6. Ibid.

7. Dr. Kenneth R. Pelletier. *Mind as Healer, Mind as Slayer*. Delta, 1978. Updated and revised edition is forthcoming.

8. Jack Dreyfus. *A Remarkable Medicine Has Been Overlooked*. Simon and Schuster, 1981. 2nd edition by Lantern Books, 2000.

9. For information on low dose Naltrexone, please visit: http://www.lowdosenaltrexone.org/.

10. "Living Longer with Heart Disease." The Noninvasive Heart Center. Article available online at: http://www.heartprotect.com/mortality-stats.shtml.

11. University of Ottawa Institute. Ontario, Canada. For statistics, including a chart representing repeat bypass surgery for three years post-op, please see: http://www.heartprotect.com/mortality-stats.shtml.

12. L. Packer. "Health Effects of Nutritional Antioxidants." 15:685–86, 1993.

T. Byers. "Vitamin E Supplements and Coronary Heart Disease." *Nutritional Review*. 50:333–45, 1993.

13. C. Norman Shealy, MD, PhD. *Holy Water, Sacred Oil: The Fountain of Youth*. Biogenics Books. 2000.

Chapter 15: Brain Chemistry Disorders

1. Michael Gershon, MD. *The Second Brain: A Groundbreaking New Understanding of Nervous Disorders of the Stomach and Intestine*. HarperCollins, 1999.

2. Ibid.

3. *See Chapter 9, Note 3.*

4. Abram Hoffer, MD, PhD. "Schizophrenia: A New Approach II. Result of a Year's Research." *Journal of Mental Science*. 100:29–45, 1954.

5. Abram Hoffer, MD, PhD. "The Vitamin Paradigm Wars." Article available online at: http://www.internetwks.com/pauling/hoffer.html.

Abram Hoffer has authored numerous books on the relationship between nutrition, orthomolecular medicine and brain chemistry. For more information, visit:

http://www.amazon.com/Abram-Hoffer/e/B001JP4PRO/ref=sr_ntt_srch_lnk_1?_encoding=UTF8&qid=1271211607&sr=1-1.

6. Alexander Schauss, PhD. *Diet, Crime and Delinquency: A New Breakthrough to Crime Control*. Parker House Enterprises, 1981.

7. William Philpott, MD. *Brain Allergies: The Psychonutrient and Magnetic Connections*. Keats, 1980. Revised and reprinted 2nd edition by McGraw-Hill, 2000.

8. Barbara Reed, PhD. *Food, Teens and Behavior*. Natural Press, 1983.

9. J. Britton, et al. "Dietary Magnesium, Lung Function, Wheezing, and Airway Hyperreactivity in a Random Sample." *Lancet*. 344–345:7–62, 1994.

S. Baker. "Magnesium in Primary Care Medicine." *Magnesium and Trace Elements*. 10:251–5, 1994.

10. M.L. Brewster and M.F. Jacobson. "The Changing American Diet." Center for Science in the Public Interest. Washington, DC., 1978.

To view the most up-to-date soft drink consumption by nation statistics, visit: http://www.nationmaster.com/graph/foo_sof_dri_con-food-soft-drink-consumption/.

11. *See Chapter 9, Note 6.*

12. *See Chapter 1, Note 12.*

Chapter 16: Arthritic Disorders

1. Taylor and Joanna Hay. *Synergetics: Your Whole Life Fitness Plan*. Pocket Books Health, 1991. *See also* DVD with the same name.

2. Michael J. Gelb. *Body Learning: An Introduction to the Alexander Technique*. Henry Holt & Co., 1981.

Lynda Huey and Robert Forster. *The Complete Waterpower Workout Book: Programs for Fitness, Injury Prevention, and Healing*. Random House, 1993.

Steven Shafarman. *Awareness Heals: The Feldenkrais Method for Dynamic Health*. Da Capo Press, 1997.

3. *See Chapter 6, Note 5.*

4. Craig Sams. "Nightshade Foods." Article available online at: http://www.organicfoodee.com/inspiration/craig/nightshadefoods/.

5. Marshall Mandell, MD. *Dr. Mandell's Lifetime Arthritis Relief System*. Berkley Publishing Group, 1985.

Theron Randolph, MD. *Environmental Medicine: Beginnings & Bibliographies of Clinical Ecology*. Clinical Ecology Publications. 1987.

6. Ibid.

7. "Seedy Remedy for Rheumatoid Arthritis?" *Science News*. 144: 302. November 6, 1993.

8. Your local chiropractor is likely an expert on quality nutritional supplements. Examples of high quality supplement manufacturers include Metagenics, Garden of Life, Standard Process, Integrative Therapeutics, Inc., Biotics Research and Nutri-West.

Chapter 17: Cancer

1. "We Are Losing the War on Cancer." *Scientific American*. January, 1994.

2. Samuel S. Epstein, MD. *The Politics of Cancer*. Reprinted as *The Politics of Cancer, Revisited*. East Ridge Press, 1998.

Ralph W. Moss, PhD. *The Cancer Industry: The Classic Expose on the Cancer Establishment*. Revised updated edition. Equinox Press, 1996.

Gary Null, PhD, et al. *Death by Medicine*, 2003. Full report available online at: http://www.whale.to/a/null9.html.

3. John W. Gofman. *Preventing Breast Cancer: The Story of a Major, Proven, Preventable Cause of This Disease*. 2nd edition. Committee for Nuclear Responsibility, 1996.

Dawn Prate. "Mammograms Cause Breast Cancer (and Other Cancer Facts You Probably Never Knew)." *Natural News*. August 15, 2005.

4. Visit the University of Chicago Comprehensive Cancer Center at: http://uccrc.uchicago.edu.

5. For more information on cancer prevention, contact the following:

1) Cancer Prevention Coalition: http://www.preventcancer.com.
2) Cancer Control Society: http://www.cancercontrolsociety.com.
3) Cancer Treatment Centers of America: http://www.cancercenter.com.

6. "Selenium Supplements Can Reduce Cancer Rate." *Science News*. Cornell University. January 7, 1997. http://uccrc.uchicago.edu.

7. Samuel S. Epstein. "American Cancer Society: The World's Wealthiest Non-Profit Institution." *International Journal of Health Services*. 29(3): 565–578, 1999.

8. *See Chapter 17, Note 5 plus:*

James S. Gordon, MD. *Comprehensive Cancer Care: Integrating Alternative, Complementary and Conventional Therapies*. Perseus, 2000.

As an additional resource, *Science News* has been reporting the latest on cancer research for the past two decades.

9. Ibid.

Chapter 18: Acne and Sebaceous Cysts

1. Leung Lit-Hung, MD. "A Stone That Kills Two Birds: Pantothenic Acid in the Treatment of Acne Vulgaris and Obesity." Article available online at: http://www.vitaminb5acne.com/study.html.

2. Leung Lit-Hung, MD. "Pantothenic Acid in the Treatment of Acne Vulgaris: 'A Medical Hypothesis'" *Journal of Orthomolecular Medicine*. 12(2), 1997. Article available online at: http://www.coenzyme-a.com/acne_vulgaris.html.

Chapter 19: Fungal Infections of the Feet

1. See "Sporonox Side Effects." and "Lamisil Side Effects." Drugs.com. Articles available online at: http://www.drugs.com/sfx/sporanox-side-effects.html and http://www.drugs.com/sfx/lamisil-side-effects.html.

2. Dr. Stoll has been recommending vinegar for toenail fungus for decades. Many testimonials can be found in the archives of his website at: http://askwaltstollmd.com/archives/toe.html.

Chapter 20: Acid Reflux (GERD)

1. Dr. Stoll's former traditional Chinese medicine (TCM) specialist first told him about ginger root juice many years ago. Since hearing of it, Dr. Stoll found that every patient who tried it reported back that they had been "cured."

Chapter 21: Constipation and Stool Withholding

1. For more information, visit The American Academy of Pediatrics at: http://www.aap.org/.

See also: Jessica Williams. "Withholding: A Common Toilet Training Challenge." *Toddlers Today*. Article available online at: http://www.toddlerstoday.com/resources/articles/withholding.htm.

2. Dr. Stoll has been recommending the fiber/mineral oil protocol for decades. Many testimonials can be found in the archives of his website at: http://askwaltstollmd.com/archives/const.html.

3. "Aspiration Pneumonitis and Pneumonia." *Merck*. May, 2008. Article available online at: http:// www.merck.com/mmpe/sec05/ch052/ch052f.html.

4. Cynthia Lair. *Feeding the Whole Family: Cooking with Whole Foods*. 3rd edition. Sasquatch Books, 2008.

Beth Loiselle. *The Healing Power of Whole Foods*. Healthways Nutrition, 1993. To be updated in 2010.

Alissa Segersten and Tom Malterre. *The Whole Life Nutrition Cookbook: Whole Foods Recipes for Personal and Planetary Health*. 2nd edition. Whole Life Press, 2007.

Chapter 22: Excessive Body Odor

1. Kimberly Shannon. "Antiperspirants: The Dangers of Sweat Prevention. November 6, 2008. Article available online at: http:// www.thebreastcancerguide.org.

2. Joel Fuhrman and Neal D. Barnard. *Fasting—and Eating—for Health: A Medical Doctor's Program for Conquering Disease*. St. Martin's Press, 1995.

Steve Meyerowitz, et al. *Juice Fasting and Detoxification: Use the Healing Power of Fresh Juice to Feel Young and Look Great: The Fastest Way to Restore Your Health*. Three Rivers Press, 1997.

Michael T. Murray. *Complete Book of Juicing: Your Delicious Guide to Youthful Vitality*. Three Rivers Press, 1997.

Chapter 23: Introduction to the 3LS

1. *See Chapter 5, Note 2.*

Chapter 24: Skilled Relaxation (The 1st Leg)

1. Herbert Benson, MD. *The Relaxation Response*. G.K. Hall, 1976. This #1 bestseller was updated, expanded, reprinted edition with co-author Miriam Z. Klipper in 2000 by Harper Paperbacks.

See also: Jess Stearn. *The Power of Alpha Thinking: Miracle of the Mind*. Signet, 1977.

2. Ibid.

3. *See Chapter 7, Note 6.*

4. Davis, et al. *The Relaxation & Stress Reduction Workbook.* 6th edition. New Harbinger Publications, 2008.

5. Eckhart Tolle. *A New Earth: Awakening to Your Life's Purpose.* Plume, 2006.

Eckhart Tolle. *The Power of Now: A Guide to Spiritual Enlightenment.* New World Library, 2004.

Eckhart Tolle. *Stillness Speaks.* New World Library, 2003.

6. *See Chapter 12, Note 4.*

7. Robert O. Becker, MD and Gary Selden. *The Body Electric: Electromagnetism and the Foundation of Life.* Harper Paperbacks, 1998.

Richard Gerber, MD. *Vibrational Medicine: The #1 Handbook of Subtle Energy Therapies.* 3rd edition. Bear & Company. 2001.

Chapter 25: Aerobic Exercise (The 2nd Leg)

1. Richard Weil. "Aerobic Exercise." Article available online at: http://www.medicinenet.com/aerobic_exercise/article.htm.

See also: Kenneth H. Cooper, MD. *The Aerobics Way.* Bantam Books. 1981.

Kathleen Ekdahl. "Understanding the Benefits of Aerobic Exercise." The New England Wellness Web. Article available online at: http://www.newellness.com/physfitn/benaero.htm.

2. Aerobics and Fitness Association of America (AFAA). *Aerobics: Theory and Practice.* AFAA, 1985.

3. *Ibid.*

4. *See Chapter 24, Note 6.*

Chapter 26: Whole Foods (The 3rd Leg)

1. AP Wire Service, 2001.

For more information, visit the National Research Council (NRC) website at: http://sites.nationalacademies.org/NRC/index.htm.

2. Paavo Airola, ND, PhD. *Are You Confused? De-Confusion Book on Nutrition & Health.* Health Plus Publishers, 1981.

Phyllis A. Balch, CNC. *Prescription for Nutritional Healing.* 4th edition. Avery Trade, 2006.

Beth Loiselle. *The Healing Power of Whole Foods.* Healthways Nutrition, 1993.

3. Ibid.

4. Ringsdorf, et al. "Sucrose, Neutrophilic Phagocytosis, and Resistance to Disease." *Dent. Surv.* 52: #12, 46–48, December, 1976.

See also: "Add Sugar, Subtract Immunity?" *USA Today.* Article available online at: http://www.usatoday.com/LIFE/usaedition/2009-10-05-bline05_ST_U.htm.

5. Ibid.

6. *See Chapter 26, Note 3 plus:* Dr. Emanuel Charaskin. *Psychodietetics: Food as the Key to Emotional Health.* Scarborough House, 1989.

Abram Hoffer, MD, PhD and Morton Walker. *Orthomolecular Nutrition: New Lifestyle for Super Good Health.* Keats Publishing, 1978. Updated, revised and reprinted as *Putting It All Together: The New Orthomolecular Nutrition.* McGraw Hill, 1998.

Harvey M. Ross, MD and Geraldine Saunders. *Hypoglycemia: The Disease Your Doctor Won't Treat.* Pinnacle, 1982. Completely revised and updated as *Hypoglycemia: The Classic Healthcare Handbook.* Kensington, 2002.

To learn more about sugar addiction, read *The End of Overeating: Taking Control of the Insatiable American Appetite* by David Kessler, MD, former head of the FDA, published in 2009 by Rodale. In addition, any online search using the keywords "sugar addiction" will return ample information and books written on the subject.

7. Beth Loiselle. *The Healing Power of Whole Foods.* Healthways Nutrition, 1993.

8. Ibid.

9. Nina Bai. "Move Over, Heroin: Sugar Addiction May Be a Reality." *Discover.* December 10, 2008.

10. *See Chapter 26, Note 7.*

Chapter 27: Elimination/Provocation Diet

1. *See Chapter 9, Note 6.*

2. *See Chapter 9, Note 6 plus:* Beth Loiselle. *The Healing Power of Whole Foods.* Healthways Nutrition, 1993. To be updated in 2011.

3. "Calcium Hydroxyapatite: The Only Form of Calcium Proven to Reverse Bone Loss." Article available online at: http://www.oralchelation.com/technical/calcium2.htm.

Dr. Deborah Baker. "Treatment for Osteoporosis-Osteopenia." Article available online at: http://y2khealthanddetox.com/Osteoporosis.htm.

Karl Loren. "What Does Your Hip Bone Look Like?" Article available online at: http://www.oralchelation.com/calcium/boneupa.htm

Further references on the efficacy of microcrystalline hydroxyapatite concentrate (MCHC) can be found here: http://www.oralchelation.com/calcium/footbone/fbscient.htm.

4. "What Grains Are Gluten-Free?" *Gluten-Free Network.* Article available online at: http://glutenfreenetwork.com/gluten-free-cooking/what-grains-are-gluten-free/.

Chapter 28: Intracellular Magnesium

1. S. Baker. "Magnesium in Primary Care Medicine." *Magnesium and Trace Elements.* 10:251–5, 1994.

J. Britton, et al. "Dietary Magnesium, Lung Function, Wheezing, and Airway Hyperreactivity in a Random Sample." *Lancet.* 344–345:7–62, 1994.

Jean Durlach, et al. *Magnesium in Cellular Processes and Medicine*. S. Karger Publishing. 1987. (See also Jean Durlach's monograph, *Magnesium in Clinical Practice*. John Libbey, 1988.)

Mildred S. Seelig, MD. *Magnesium Requirements in Human Nutrition*. Karger, 1987.

2. Ibid.

3. Norman C. Shealy, MD, PhD. *Holy Water, Sacred Oil: The Fountain of Youth*. Biogenics Books, 2000.

4. *See Chapter 8, Note 3.*

5. Ancient Minerals Ultra Pure Topical Magnesium Products. http://www.ancient-minerals.com.

Chapter 29: Essential Fatty Acids

1. Y. Mardens, et al. "GC-MS Profiling of Urinary Organic Acids Evaluated as a Quantitative Method." *Clinical Chemistry*. 42:1609–15, 1996.

M.T. Clandinin, et al. "Normal Subjects Consuming Physiological Levels of 18:3 (n-3) and 20:5 (n-3) from Flaxseed or Fish Oils Have Characteristic Differences in Plasma Lipid and Lipoprotein Fatty Acid Levels." *Journal of Nutrition*. 126:2130–40, 1996.

J.R. Burgess, et al. "Omega-3 Fatty Acids in Boys with Behavior, Learning and Health Problems." *Physiological Behavior*. 59:915–20, 1996.

Fifteen additional educational articles and research studies on EFAs can be found at: http://www.barleans.com/literature.asp.

2. For more information on selecting high-qualtity supplements including independent test results, visit ConsumerLab.com.

Chapter 30: Avoiding Unnecessary Antibiotics

1. *Journal of Clinical Microbiology*. 36:539–542, 1998.

See also: Chapter 11, Note 1.

Alan Green, MD. "Antibiotic Overuse." Article available online at: http://www.drgreene.com/qa/antibiotic-overuse.

2. Steve Baragona. "U.S. Antibiotic Use in Livestock Harms People." Voice of America. Article available online at: http://www.voanews.com/english/news/usa/US-Antibiotic-Use-in-Livestock-Harms-People-98921789.html.

3. Darryl C. Tong, BDS, MSD. "Antibiotic Prophylaxis in Dentistry: A Review and Practice Recommendations." *The Journal of the American Dental Assocation*. Article available online at: http://jada.ada.org/cgi/content/full/131/3/366.

Chapter 32: Gentle Rebounding

1. Albert E. Carter. *The New Miracles of Rebound Exercise*. Nature Distributors. 1988.

See also: Albert E. Carter. *Rebound Exercise: The Ultimate Exercise for the New Millennium*. AuthorHouse, 2005.

Sandy Halliday. "Speed Up Your Detox with Mini Trampoline Exercises." The Detox Specialist. Article available online at: http://thedetoxspecialist.com/blog/detox/speed-up-your-detox-with-mini-trampoline-exercises.

Bente Hewitt. "Rebounding: A Great Way to Detox Your Body." SelfGrowth.com. Article available online at: http://www.selfgrowth.com/articles/Rebounding_A_Great_Way_to_Detox_your_Body.html.

2. Ibid.

3. Edgar Cayce's Association for Research & Enlightenment (A.R.E.). http://edgarcayce.org/.

Information about Cayce's castor oil remedy can be found here: http://edgarcaycediet.com/Articles/castor_oil_packs.htm.

Information on coffee enemas can be found here: http://www.naturalhealthtechniques.com/HealingTechniques/Enemas.htm#Coffee_enemas/.

Information on liver and gallbladder cleansing can be found here: http://www.astrodreamadvisor.com/Body_Apple_Fast.html and here: http://edgarcayceonline.com/eco/Karma-Cleanse.aspx.

Chapter 33: Applied Kinesiology

1. Donna Eden, et al. *Energy Medicine*. Tarcher, 1999.

John Diamond, MD. *Your Body Doesn't Lie*. Grand Central Publishing, 1989.

See also: Susan L. Levy and Carol Lehr. *Your Body Can Talk: How to Use Simple Muscle Testing to Learn What Your Body Knows and Needs*. Hohm Press, 1996.

John Lepore, ND. *The Ultimate Healing System: The Illustrated Guide to Muscle Testing and Nutrition*. Woodland Publishin, 1998.

Appendix A: The Doctor-Patient Relationship

1. Charles B. Inlander and Eugene I. Pavalon. *Your Medical Rights: How to Become an Empowered Consumer*. 2nd edition. People's Medical Society, 1994.

David Stutz, MD and Benard Feder, PhD. *The Savvy Patient: How to Be an Active Participant in Your Medical Care*. Consumer Reports Books, 1990.

Acknowledgments for Walt Stoll, MD

1. *See Chapter 1, Note 12.*

2. *See Introduction, Note 1.*

Glossary

Most terms are clearly defined within the text of the book. For definitions not found here, please see the extensive glossary available on Dr. Stoll's website: http://askwaltstollmd.com/glossary.php.

acute illness: Any illness that comes on suddenly, is self-limited and short-lived. Conventional medical treatment can be a helpful option for acute illnesses. See also **chronic illness.**

Aerobic Exercise: Any type of non-strenuous, sustained, large-muscle exercise activity that consistently maintains the heart rate within a specific target range for a minimum of 12½ minutes.

allergy: A condition in which a substance from the environment stimulates serum antibodies in the blood, causing an inappropriate immune response. See also **hypersensitivity.**

allopathic medicine: The atomistic healing philosophy commonly known today as "conventional medicine." See also **conventional medicine** and **atomism.**

alpha: A brain wave frequency of between 8–12 cycles per second (cps). The state of alpha or theta must be reached for the practice of Skilled Relaxation to be successful. See also **relaxation response.**

alternative medicine: A general term referring to any healing philosophy or technique other than conventional medicine.

amino acids: Small molecules that combine to form peptides, which then combine to form proteins via peptide bonds. Amino acids are typically defined as the "building blocks of protein." See also **peptides.**

anthroposophical medicine: A vitalistic healing philosophy based on the teachings of Rudolph Steiner. It includes theosophy with a focus on attaining the wisdom of the spiritual world.

antibiotic: A general term for medications designed to kill specific susceptible bacteria in an acute bacterial infection. Antibiotics are generally over-used, and are ineffective against viral infections.

antibody: A specific-shaped immunoglobin which binds with and neutralizes an antigen. See also **antigen.**

antigen: A substance that the immune system considers to be an invader (bacteria, viruses, toxins, etc.) and so attempts to neutralize it by creating a specifically shaped antibody. See also **antibody.**

antioxidant: A chemical compound or substance (such as vitamins C, E and beta carotene) that protects body cells from the damage of oxidation by neutralizing free radicals. See also **free radical.**

applied kinesiology (AK): A diagnostic system that uses "muscle testing" to receive information from the bodymind about whether a certain food or substance might be helpful or harmful to an individual.

atherosclerosis: A condition characterized by clogging of the arteries with cholesterol plaques in the intima (the stretchy lining of the arteries right under the endothelium—the one-cell thick internal lining of the arteries).

atomism: The philosophy that the human bodymind is nothing more than a "machine" in which tiny particles get combined and recombined. Atomism is the basis for the allopathic paradigm as we know it today. See also **vitalism.**

ayurvedic medicine: A vitalistic healing philosophy based on the ancient Hindu science of health and medicine, which focuses on assisting the body to heal itself—the antithesis of the allopathic philosophy.

beta: A brain-wave frequency of 13 or more cycles per second (cps). This is the normal, awake, thinking brain-wave rhythm.

biofeedback training: A process in which, using an electronic monitoring device, an individual learns to reliably influence the physiological responses of the body (breathing, body temperature, heart rate and blood pressure). See also **Skilled Relaxation.**

bodymind: A term which illustrates that the body and the mind are not separate or independent of one another, and that each affects the other.

bracing: A condition of unconscious, total-body chronic muscle tension due to severe, overwhelming stored stress-effect in the hypothalamus.

Candida-related syndrome (C-RS): The fungal form of a parasitic organism called Candida albicans, typically invading the intestinal tract after LGS is present. See also **leaky gut syndrome.**

casein: A type of protein present in milk and several other dairy products. Casein and gluten are the two most common food proteins responsible for unidentified hypersensitivity reactions in many people, not detected by conventional allergy testing. See also **gluten** and **hypersensitivity.**

chiropractic medicine: A vitalistic healing philosophy specializing in the science and art of the interrelationship between the musculoskeletal system and the various functions of the body.

chronic illness: Any illness or set of symptoms that develops slowly, remains persistent over a long period of time or is recurring. Chronic conditions are not well managed by and typically cannot be cured by conventional medicine. See also **acute illness.**

complementary medicine: Alternative medicine used in conjunction with (as a complement to) conventional medicine.

congenital: Refers to any gene-related condition existing at the time of birth (in fact, present from the moment of conception).

conventional medicine: The atomistic healing philosophy that operates as a powerful functional monopoly in the U.S. Its forte is acute conditions. For chronic conditions, however, its emphasis is on treating the symptoms of illness rather than prevention and curing at the cause. Also known as **allopathic medicine** and **atomism.**

cure: To heal a condition permanently, usually by eliminating its root cause. Often erroneously used interchangeable with the word "treatment." See also **treatment.**

delta: A brain wave frequency of less than 4 cycles per second (cps). Delta is the state of sleep, and is also the point at which loss of muscle control occurs. Some highly experienced Zen masters are able to maintain delta while awake during meditation.

diagnosis: The formal name for a particular health condition, given by a medical doctor, according to your symptoms and/or laboratory test results. Often, it is an educated guess.

dis-ease: A way of spelling "disease" to emphasize that it means not being at ease.

disease care: The conventional medical monopoly's approach to treating disease based on symptom suppression. A disease-care approach lacks patient education in prevention, lifestyle and Wellness. See also **health care.**

double-blind study: A testing procedure designed to eliminate biased results by ensuring that neither the tester nor the one being tested knows what treatment is being given until the end of the study. See also **placebo effect.**

dysautonomia: Dysfunction of the autonomic nervous system due to severe, prolonged stress-effect storage in the hypothalamus.

dysbiosis: An imbalance of the normal bacterial population (flora) of the gut and degradation of a healthy intestinal ecology.

electromagnetic soup: A term to denote the "thick" atmosphere of electromagnetic radiation (given off by power lines, radio waves, electric clocks and blankets, TV and computer screens, etc.) all of which are stressors to the bodymind.

essential fatty acids (EFAs): Essential types of oils that cannot be made within the body and so must be obtained from the environment (diet). Basically, EFAs are "fat vitamins."

fight-or-flight (FOF) response: A term coined by Dr. Hans Selye to denote the primitive life-saving internal response to real or perceived danger. One of its natural purposes is to supply adrenaline to prepare the body for the strength and/or endurance for fighting or fleeing. It is the most basic of the stress responses of any organism (even an amoeba has it).

free radical: A highly reactive atom or group of atoms with an unpaired electron. Free radicals have damaging effects on the body when not paired with antioxidants. See also **antioxidant.**

gluten: A type of protein present in some grains such as wheat, rye and barley. Gluten and casein are the two most common food proteins that are responsible for unidentified hypersensitivity reactions in many people, not detected by conventional allergy testing. See also **casein** and **hypersensitivity.**

gut: The intestinal tract, which happens to be one long continuous tube from mouth to anus.

health care (the true meaning): A healing approach that gives the patient complete freedom and access to whatever healing philosophy is best suited for his or her condition, as well as a holistic focus on the prevention and elimination of the root causes of disease via a Wellness lifestyle. See also **disease care.**

Hellerwork: A specific method of deep-tissue structural bodywork and movement education designed to re-align the body and release chronic tension and stress.

histamine: A chemical released by the body during an allergic reaction, causing runny nose, sneezing, itching, rashes or anaphylaxis.

holistic medicine: A vitalistic healing philosophy that emphasizes seeing the person as a whole, focusing on education and responsible lifestyle choices to achieve balance and well-being. Holistic medicine, by definition, encompasses the effective components of *all* the world's healing philosophies, including conventional medicine.

homeopathic medicine: A vitalistic healing philosophy based on stimulating your body's own inner healing ability through minute doses of safe substances based on a principle of "like cures like."

hypersensitivity: A condition in which peptides leak through the gut wall stimulating cellular antibodies, causing an immune response. Two common examples are milk protein (casein) and wheat protein (gluten). Since tissue hypersensitivities cannot be detected by conventional serum allergy testing, most people are unaware of this mechanism as the cause of their symptoms. See also **allergy.**

hypothalamus: A small region of the brain that controls many bodily functions and is the connection between the brain and the body as far as hormones and metabolism are concerned. The hypothalamus is home to accumulated stress-effect storage, which can be discharged through the regular practice of effective Skilled Relaxation in order to reverse the root cause of chronic health conditions.

immune system: The complex network of organs, tissues, molecules and cells whose job it is to defend the body against unwanted invaders, such as bacteria, viruses, fungi and parasites.

leaky gut syndrome (LGS): A condition in which the lining of the intestinal tract (gut) has become permeable (leaky) and is no longer sufficiently protecting the inner body from foreign substances. See also **gut.**

mineral: A substance that is neither animal nor vegetable, an inorganic element essential to the nutrition of humans, animals and plants.

molecular medicine: The science of determining abnormal function at the level of molecules rather than waiting until entire organs malfunction.

monopoly: The exclusive possession or control of a group over a commodity or service.

naturopathic medicine: A vitalistic healing philosophy based on combining the use of natural substances with supporting the innate healing capacity of the bodymind.

osteopathic medicine: A healing philosophy based on treating the whole person instead of just the symptoms, with an appreciation of the body's ability to heal itself. Doctors of osteopathy (DOs) have at least the equivalent conventional medical licensing as MDs, yet they combine this atomistic practice with vitalistic approaches.

paradigm: A way of viewing reality based on a set of concepts, values and assumptions. Some paradigms, though they may be false, are strongly held by entire communities of people.

peptides: Portion of food proteins, not fully broken down, containing a chain of at least three amino acids. See also **amino acids.**

pituitary: Formerly considered the "master gland" of the endocrine system, the pituitary gland influences the function of all the other endocrine glands. It is located beneath the hypothalamus at the base of the brain.

placebo effect: An effect, typically beneficial but sometimes negative, that arises from the patient's belief in a treatment, even if that "treatment" is nothing but water in a syringe or a sugar pill. See also **double-blind study.**

probiotic: A term used to denote microorganisms that are considered healthy or beneficial to the body. For example, Lactobacillus acidophilus and Bifidobacterium populations in the gut.

psychosocial: Pertaining to the psychological development of the individual in relation to his or her social environment.

"quack": A doctor who is untrained, ignorant or dispenses what is considered to be dangerous medical advice or treatment. This term is commonly slung at any conventional practitioner who dares to begin incorporating complementary healing modalities over the past century.

refined carbohydrate: Any carbohydrate that has been stripped of its covering, its "germ," its peel or its pulp, so that it no longer contains within itself, as a living food, all the elements—vitamins, minerals, proteins, enzymes, fiber—necessary for metabolizing itself or being metabolized.

relaxation response: A special state of mind consisting of a preponderance of "alpha" or "theta" brain-wave frequencies, which is the goal of effective Skilled Relaxation. See also **Skilled Relaxation.**

Rolfing: Named after Ida Rolf, Rolfing is a holistic system of structural/psychological integration involving deep soft-tissue manipulation for bringing the head, neck, torso, pelvis, legs and feet into balance.

Skilled Relaxation (SR): The 20-minute, twice-a-day practice of any technique that brings about the relaxation response in you. With faithful practice, SR helps reverse chronic health conditions at their root cause by discharging stored stress-effect in the hypothalamus. See also **relaxation response** and **biofeedback.**

stress: Defined by Dr. Hans Selye as "the nonspecific response of the body to any demand." Stress can be thought of as anything that requires the body to adapt. See also **stress-effect.**

stress-effect: The fight-or-flight response, which when not immediately discharged through the act of physically fighting or fleeing, becomes stored in the hypothalamus. While short-term stress response is good for the bodymind, in most cases, the overwhelming burden of the accumulation of stress-effect storage is the root cause of most chronic conditions. See also **fight-or-flight response** and **hypothalamus.**

symptom: An outward sign of the existence of an underlying condition, such as pain, bleeding, itching, fatigue, etc. Treating symptoms with medications without addressing the underlying cause is the equivalent of putting tape over the warning lights on your dashboard, or cutting the wires to the doorbell so you cannot hear your neighbor trying to tell you that your house is on fire.

theta: A brain wave frequency of between 4–8 cycles per second (cps). The state of alpha or theta must be reached for the practice of Skilled Relaxation to be successful. See also **relaxation response.**

traditional Chinese medicine (TCM): A vitalistic healing philosophy that utilizes nutrition, herbs, acupuncture, massage and Qigong.

treatment: Any of a number of remedies intended to alleviate the symptoms of an acute or chronic illness, injury or disease. No treatment can cure a chronic health condition. See also **cure.**

vitalism: The philosophy that the human bodymind has within it the capacity to protect itself from environmental degradations and aging. All healing philosophies of the world, except allopathy, are based in vitalism. See also **atomism.**

Wellness: More than the absence of disease, Wellness is a state of being in which body, mind and spirit are healthy and in harmony with each other and the environment.

Whole Food: A food that is in its natural state containing all its nutrient-rich living parts, without having been processed or refined in any way.

Index

Asterisks indicate notes located at the bottom of that page.
Italicized page numbers indicate graphs and illustrations.
For definitions of terms, please see the Glossary.

C

D

E

F

G

H

I

N

S

T

X

Y

Z

About the Authors

Walt Stoll, MD

Walt is a holistic health educator who was in practice for more than thirty years as a board-certified family practitioner. He was a founding member of the American Holistic Medical Association (AHMA), and the last seventeen years of his thirty-year career were spent practicing holistic medicine.

In 1996, Walt wrote and published his first book, *Saving Yourself from the Disease-Care Crisis*. In 2006, he co-authored and published the award-winning book, *Recapture Your Health*. He is the medical director of the Stoll Foundation for Holistic Health, and host of the popular website "Ask Dr. Stoll" (www.askwaltstollmd.com), where he has answered health questions free of charge for the past fifteen years.

Kathleen M. Diehl

Kathleen is a writer, editor and awareness-based spiritual coach with over eighteen years of personal study and formal training in a variety of spiritual, metaphysical, holistic and alternative health philosophies. She has authored several articles on awareness-based living, and has been a featured guest on two radio shows.

In 2009, Kathleen wrote and published her first book, *The Collective Awakening*. To learn more about spiritual awakening, awareness and personal evolution, or for more information on her website editing and book proofreading services, please visit her website at www.kathleendiehl.com.

9310886R0

Made in the USA
Charleston, SC
31 August 2011